Cancer is not just a ¡ emotionally and spiritual. ... ~~, ...~~ ~~.. /~~ ~~...~~.. *Dr. Sealy's book is an honest and open account of a woman and her family's struggle with cancer. The journaling of her own passion story in terms of Christ's passion has a long history in Christian spirituality. I have no doubt that Pat's story will resonate emotionally and spiritually with other cancer sufferers, their families and care givers. The reflections at the end of each chapter are insightful, helpful, and thought provoking. Dr. Sealy's story is a courageous journey from death to life—through pain and suffering to hope—by a cancer survivor who has discovered a deeper appreciation and understanding of life.*
—Rev. Dr. David McKane

A heartfelt story of a family's journey with breast cancer. It is filled with hope, love and courage. Dr. Sealy has has given voice to the family crisis and adaptation through her spouse Kevin's Peaceable Kingdom, *daughter Eliza's* Invincible *(age 14), daughter Leonie's* A Scary Thought *(age 10), long-term friend Karen's* Adversity Story, *and Rev. Kate Hathaway's* A Journey with Pat Sealy. *This book celebrates the marriage of nursing, Christian and spiritual practices.*
—Dale Rajacich RN, PhD Associate Professor

A FAMILY'S RESURRECTION FROM
BRE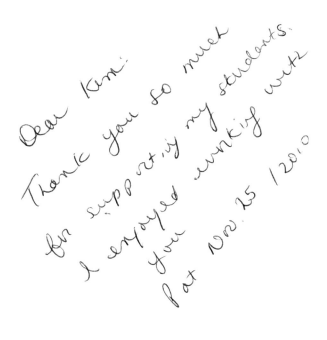ST CANCER

PATRICIA A. SEALY, R.N., Ph.D.

Dear Kim:
Thank you so much
for supporting my students.
I enjoyed working with
you
Pat Nov 25 /2010

Guardian BOOKS

Belleville, Ontario, Canada

A FAMILY'S RESURRECTION FROM BREAST CANCER
Copyright © 2010, Patricia Sealy

Scripture quotations marked NIV are taken from the HOLY BIBLE, NEW INTERNATIONAL VERSION ®. Copyright © 1973, 1978, 1984 by International Bible Society. Used by permission of Zondervan Publishing House. All rights reserved. • Scripture quotations marked KJV are taken from *The Holy Bible, King James Version.* Copyright © 1977, 1984, Thomas Nelson Inc., Publishers.

ISBN: 978-1-55452-561-4
LSI Edition: 978-1-55452-562-1

To order additional copies, visit:
www.essencebookstore.com

For more information, please contact:
Patricia Sealy
7-1615 North Routledge Park
London, ON N6H 5L6
www.patsealybreastca.ca

Guardian Books is an imprint of *Essence Publishing,* a Christian Book Publisher dedicated to furthering the work of Christ through the written word. For more information, contact:
20 Hanna Court, Belleville, Ontario, Canada K8P 5J2
Phone: 1-800-238-6376 • Fax: (613) 962-3055
E-mail: info@essence-publishing.com
Web site: www.essence-publishing.com

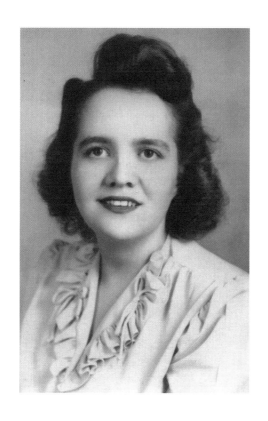

In Memoriam

Jean Elizabeth Sealy (Bell)

December 27, 1921

May 13, 1961

Better to remember and weep,

Than to repress and be fearful.

No longer lost, but found.

Acknowledgements

I can in all sincerity say, "Thank God I'm alive."

I am very grateful to my husband, Kevin Webb, and my daughters Eliza and Leonie for surviving my breast cancer with me.

I would like to thank Dr. Potvin (Chemotherapy Oncologist), Dr. Holiday (Surgeon), Pat Baruth (Nurse Practitioner), Dr. Pereira (Radiation Oncologist), Dr. Powers (Gynecologist/Endocrinologist) and Dr. Kumar (Family Practitioner) and Joanne Pack (Registered Massage Therapist) for their caring and concern during my treatment and recovery.

I would like to thank my friends Karen Adamson, Kate Hathaway, Lesley Bell, Jodi Dunn, and Elaine Vincent for continuously supporting me through my treatment and recovery. I would also like to thank my nephew Mike and niece Michelle and their children Livvey and Jilly for being there for me. I am very grateful my sister Jean moved to London from Michigan to London.

I would like to thank Helen Battler, Rev. Kate Hathaway and Rev. Mona Goulette for their spiritual support as well as Deborah Carter who led our meditation group along with its members for all of their support.

I would like to thank Charlene Beynon, Ashley Hoogenboom and Gayle Riedl from the Middlesex-London Health Unit for supporting me while I continued to work.

I have been very fortunate to have so many people to care for and about me during my illness. I wish there was space to include all of your names.

Altogether, you have saved my life so that I have another chance to live and make a contribution in life.

Table of Contents

A Scary Thought
Leonie, Age Nine

One day I had a scary thought. My mom came into my room. I had a bad feeling inside. She said she had cancer. It gave me a terrible thought that she was going to die. I know it's a bad thought, that is why it's the title of this chapter.

She had to go through chemotherapy. It was hard for me and my sister. Almost every night I would be in my bed crying, but I kept on telling myself that it was going to be okay.

The hardest day was when my mom had the surgery. I skipped school that day.

My teacher helped me a lot through that year. Her name is Mrs. M. She is a really nice teacher. I also knew a person that I could go to when I had something on my mind. His name was Mr. H. or Steve.

A lot of people were there for me. I just didn't know that at the time, and I was scared for a very long eight months.

I missed a lot of school in the beginning, about five weeks of school. It's a lot.

I had a lot of friends that could also help me through this. It was a little hard to do all the stuff that I missed. One of my friends was going through a harder time than me.

My mom had to stay in the hospital for the whole March break because she did not feel good after the surgery. It was scary but not as much as the surgery.

If this happens to someone that you really love and is important to you, the thing to do is not worry too much because being sad doesn't help. I had to learn that the hard way, and if there's a counsellor at your school, go and talk to them. It helps. I did that because I had it all bottled up inside and that was not good, and when it came time to talk, it was harder to get me to speak.

The chemo was the hardest too. If you have someone who is special to you that has cancer, follow some of these tips because they really help.

They End (Freudian Slip)

Introduction

I have been afraid of dying my whole life. I came by this fear honestly as a result of my mother dying of acute pancreatitis when I was five years old. The age of five is a time of magical thinking, and I have suffered many consequences as a result of such a loss at that time in my life. Our family never talked about my mother's death, and I am not sure that any of us really grieved her loss openly. For me, what perhaps should have been grief came out instead as severe loneliness and pronounced anxiety. After my mother's death, I was raised by my grandfather until he died when I was ten years old. My grandpa's death completely cemented my fear of dying, perhaps for life.

I am a registered nurse, and I graduated with a Bachelor of Science in Nursing and a Bachelor of Arts degree from the University of Windsor in 1979. Upon graduating, I decided to work and travel, and I held numerous positions as a front-line nurse in Texas and Australia. Upon my return from Australia, I attended graduate school and completed my Masters in Nursing degree from the University of Western Ontario in 1987. Subsequently I worked as a nursing director in psychiatry. I have found that taking university degrees were a constant source of affirmation for me, so in 1993, I began my PhD in sociology part time (while continuing to work full time and raise my family). After a stressful nine years, I graduated in 2002. I really felt I had succeeded in life when I was fortunate enough to be hired as Nurse Researcher/Educator for the public health unit that also allowed me to teach family nursing at The University of Western Ontario.

In spite of these successes, I still carried my childhood fears and anxieties. I hid my fears from the world with the exception of my husband and close friends. I have known all of my life that the outward impression of functioning does not necessarily mean the person is not experiencing tremendous anxiety and suffering on a mental, emotional and spiritual level. I have survived many major and minor crises in my life, but for our family, breast cancer was the biggest hurdle we had ever faced. Having cancer was not just a physical and emotional crisis for our family, it was also a spiritual crisis as well. My constant lament was "Isn't it enough to be going through treatment for breast cancer, without everything else going wrong?" Kevin, Eliza and Leonie felt the same way about other issues in their lives. We were traumatized individually and collectively. It seemed that we struggled every minute.

This book originally began as a personal journal to help me acknowledge what was good and what was insightful through our experience of treatment, rather than dwelling on what was bad. I decided to write a book to help nursing students because, even though I was teaching students how to interact with families during transitions, I discovered the lived experience of breast cancer gave me a greater understanding of what is needed. There is a major clinical component to this book as I describe in detail the physical suffering during treatment. I have also shared my hopes and fears and even a few dreams to provide you with more intimate glimpse of our struggle with advanced breast cancer. In hindsight, the treatment obstacles were minor in comparison with recovery. I found it amazing that even though just about everyone I knew thought I was courageous, my fears and anxieties always made me think I was a coward; I thought I was an impostor. Whenever someone said to me that being optimistic would improve my chances of survival, I cringed inside and thought I was a "goner." Thus I have included my reflections and suggestions on how to improve nursing practice at the end of each chapter. These are the things I will tell my students when I return to teaching.

As time passed, the reason for writing the book expanded and I wanted to write it in a manner that would be understandable to anyone who has breast cancer and for their struggling family and friends. Even though there are similarities, each family's experience with cancer is unique. Some of my story may resonate with someone's personal story of breast cancer or that of a loved one. It may also resonate for people who have experienced chemotherapy, surgery or radiation for other types of cancer. We live in a world of comparisons. All the time, through treatment and recovery, I was aware that some people had it much better than me and some people had it much worse. Comparisons only make one feel better or worse in the moment. We all want to make sense of cancer in our lives from "Why me," to "Why not me," to "What is next?"

I struggled over the theme of this book. I wanted it to be more than just a story of my clinical (physical and emotional) trials and tribulations. Even more important than my personal experience, I wanted to emphasize that my family and friends also struggled daily with my cancer. We all experienced the cancer, its treatments and recovery in very different ways. Thus I felt it was important for my husband, my daughters and my friends to share their unique perspectives in this book. Everyone in my family has changed because of this journey with breast cancer. Some, like me, have experienced radical changes; others perhaps are now more sensitive to the suffering of others.

It was during one of my regular meditation sessions that I knew the title of this book would be "A Family's Resurrection from Breast Cancer." I wanted to emphasize the female and family face of suffering. I believe Jesus' passion story is the best example of male suffering, but I do not think the Gospels tell us much information about how Jesus and his family (his mother and disciples) were feeling through his terrible ordeal. I began thinking more and more about the meaning of our family's day-to-day journey of suffering, forgiveness and resurrection in relation to Maundy Thursday, Good Friday, Easter Saturday and Easter Sunday. In the end, I decided I also wanted to share a spiritual and pastoral care message.

I know our family will be terribly exposed to the world as we share the intimate details of our experience with breast cancer, through treatment and recovery. I am hoping that you, the reader, will not judge us harshly as we describe how we "fell apart" and then recovered. Leonie, my nine-year-old daughter, wrote the opening of the book, "A Scary Thought." My experiences before the diagnosis of locally advanced breast cancer and the period of diagnostic testing to discover the extent of the cancer are included in the chapter titled "In the Wilderness and Gethsemane." The period of cancer treatment (chemotherapy, double mastectomy and radiation) is included under "Good Friday." I consider the "Easter Saturday: In the Tomb" chapter to be the most important chapter, because it describes the arduous period of recovery when I was full of doubt about survival. Eliza, my fourteen-year-old daughter, wrote three sections: "Invincible" about her loss of naiveté upon discovering my cancer diagnosis, as well as "Personal Power" and "Moment of Happiness." My husband, Kevin Webb, wrote about his struggle supporting our family and his emotional growth during this period in "The Peaceable Kingdom." Karen Adamson, my best friend of forty years wrote a chapter entitled "Adversity Story" to discuss how my cancer affected her. Rev. Kate Hathaway, an Anglican priest and my friend wrote "A Journey with Pat Sealy" to describe her pastoral support for me. The book ends with my "Easter Sunday Reflections" in which I endeavoured to share my profound sense of resurrection after over twenty months of suffering and reflections as a researcher/educator, sociologist, nurse, friend, wife, mother, woman, victim, anxious person and spiritual person.

Kate tells me my story may help others to share their suffering with family, friends, clinicians and pastoral care workers, so they may find healing. Families that experience cancer need to be affirmed in their journey so that they do not feel so alone in the wilderness of their struggle. My hope is that our story will help bring comfort and help you and the people you love know you are not alone on this journey. If you find the story overwhelming in parts, go to the concluding chapter and read "Easter Sunday Reflections." This chapter will provide you with a more optimistic viewpoint and a different sense of meaning from suffering.

Overall, I think that the main messages are:

* Many people enter a life-threatening illness carrying unresolved traumas from the past.

* Cancer affected the whole family. We fell down together, and we were very fortunate to heal together even stronger.

* Breast cancer was a vehicle to understand the female and family face of suffering using the Easter passion paradigm.

* Spiritual care helped us heal from the physical and the emotional cancer in our lives.

* Because life can be very unfair, we hope our story will provide inspiration so that some good can come from suffering.

Chapter 1

In the Wilderness and Gethsemane

Jesus knew that to fulfill the scriptures he needed to experience pain and suffering on the cross. I imagine that being human, he felt tremendous trepidation knowing what was coming. The analogy of Maundy Thursday and Gethsemane fits as a model for our family's journey in the sense of knowing that something difficult or even terrible is coming and you are powerless to stop it. Many prayers are said hoping to avoid the inevitable, while feeling in your soul the pain and suffering will still come. Much of this part of the story is about the clinical waiting time, hoping that the pain would disappear.

In the Wilderness: My Experiences Before the Diagnosis

The story of Jesus in the wilderness is about self-searching and temptation. My time of self-searching was about my fears of terminal cancer and my desperate hope it wouldn't happen.

It is very easy to remember my story before the diagnosis of breast cancer because I wonder whether I will ruminate over this time period the rest of my life. I think most people with a serious illness review the prior events to see if they could have done anything differently, if they had the opportunity to relive those days. Even though I do not rationally think that something I did caused the cancer or that maybe I could have done something to aid in early diagnosis of cancer, I still find myself reviewing this period wondering *If only I....*

It was three days after Christmas 2007 when I felt some pain in the lower right section of my right breast, where the bra wire was located. I wondered if my bra was just too tight. I changed bras, but the uncomfortable feeling continued. Naturally I thought about breast cancer because I had three cysts in the right breast over the previous two years that I worried were breast cancer. Each time I had mammograms and/or ultrasounds I was reassured that they were "only cysts; your breasts are very dense" so I just thought *Here I go again.*

Having a lump in your breast can lead to a compulsive urge to constantly feel whether the lump has changed; always hoping that it has miraculously disappeared. No, it was still there. By New Year's Eve, I had probably felt the lump a hundred times. Therefore, I decided to make an appointment with Dr. Kumar, my family doctor, so I could stop being so neurotic. I really wanted to stop worrying.

Dr. Kumar made an appointment for a mammogram that was scheduled for the end of January, 2008. Since I had been down this road before, an appointment was made for an ultrasound of the breast at the end of February. I also scheduled a reappointment with Dr. Kumar at the end of January to review my progress. Unfortunately, I had to miss the latter appointment because a family friend, Mr. Red[1] (the man who actually saved me from drowning when I was a child) lay dying. It was a heartbreaking and exhausting time. I left my family on a cold wintry night to be with Mr. Red, who was living in a nursing home a two-hour drive away. I arrived at midnight and stayed awake all night to be there for him so Mrs. Red could get some sleep. All through the night, I continued to feel the lump and pain in my breast. I knew Mr. Red was dying and thought I might be dying as well. I prayed for God to bring comfort to Mr. Red; I prayed for God to relieve me of my own fear of dying prematurely. Because they had enough to deal with, I didn't tell the Reds about my fears. Mr. Red died four days later, and I came home exhausted. I went to the mammogram appointment after Mr. Red's funeral.

I was worried when I had the mammogram because I was anticipating bad news. To my surprise, the results of the mammogram were that my breasts were still very dense and that there were no changes. Even though I felt tremendous relief at not having cancer, I still had this nagging doubt that something was wrong because the pain was still there when I touched the lump. At the end of February, 2008, I went for my ultrasound appointment. My anxiety started to increase because the technician was taking longer than normal to complete the test. I interpreted the need for additional time as being the result of something serious being wrong with my breast. It felt like the ultrasound seemed to take forever to complete. After the test was completed, the radiologist came and used the ultrasound equipment herself to examine my breast. In our discussions, I told her I had had very bad mastitis (inflammation of the breast) when I was breast-feeding my daughter thirteen years before. The radiologist thought I had chronic mastitis and that it would resolve on its own. I went home jubilant and said a prayer of thanks to God for sparing me.

I continued to have the same minor pain in my breast over the next few months and kept wondering how long it would take the mastitis to heal. By June, I also noticed that my nipple was beginning to hurt as well. It felt like a blocked milk duct, similar to what I felt when I breastfed my daughter. By July, I could feel fluid in a capsule in my breast and that there was a hard lump under the fluid. The lump was really becoming painful most of the time, and I was also having pain in my right shoulder blade, so I went back to my family doctor. Dr. Kumar prescribed an antibiotic and an anti-inflammatory drug. After taking the medication for a week, the fluid portion went down but the hard lump was still there. I was pleased when Dr. Kumar made an appointment with a surgeon to deal with the mastitis. I thought the surgeon would be able to take a biopsy and find the proper antibiotic to finally take the mastitis away. Unfortunately my appointment was not until the middle of September, because my surgeon was going on vacation and there are waiting times to see a surgeon when one's previous mammogram and ultrasound are negative.

I was so tired in August. Even when I was on vacation at a cottage, I slept every afternoon and still felt very tired. After our vacation, I returned to Dr. Kumar because I thought the lump was growing. Dr. Kumar encouraged me to call the surgeon, Dr. Holiday, to try and move up the appointment. The very next day my breast started to swell. Dr. Holiday moved up the appointment to September 2, 2008. That weekend, Kevin and I went to urgent care to see if there was anything else I could do. The emergency doctor made a referral for another mammogram!

In the Garden of Gethsemane

The Garden of Gethsemane is about knowing that you are travelling down a road that you cannot change. You go with family and friends to pray and find out they have fallen asleep. Maybe your family and friends deny that terrible things are about to happen. You may have support around you, but you still feel very much alone. You pray the burden will be taken from you if possible.

I was surprised and grateful when the radiology department called and told me my appointment was for the upcoming Thursday (August 28, 2008). I expected that I would be waiting at least a couple of weeks for the mammogram. I went to the breast screening clinic at the hospital as scheduled for the mammogram. After the radiologist checked the preliminary results, the technician came back and said they would like to complete the ultrasound that afternoon. Being a nurse, I knew something was wrong when the next test was being scheduled right away. I knew they were shifting other women around to accommodate me. While I was waiting to have the ultrasound, I became more aware of the women entering the room for breast biopsies. I felt scared.

The technician brought me into the ultrasound room, and I was positioned for the test. The ultrasound gel felt warm, which was a benefit because cold ultrasound gel is a very unpleasant feeling on your breast. Just like the past February, I once again thought the technician was taking too long to complete the ultrasound. I explained to her that I had been under a great deal of stress since January because of my fear the lump was cancerous. After the ultrasound was completed, the technician left to have the radiologist review the results. I was so anxious. The radiologist

23

returned with the technician to tell me that I most likely had a neoplasm (a scientific word meaning breast cancer). The radiologist told me I could either have a biopsy immediately, or I would have to wait for the next available appointment, which was in three weeks. I felt hysterical, but thought that I couldn't handle the anxiety of waiting three additional weeks. Tasting bile in my throat, I agreed to the procedure.

I wanted to take a sedative before the biopsy to relieve my anxiety, but I had no such luck since I didn't have them with me. The radiologist injected the local anesthetic, and the biopsy was completed using the ultrasound machine. The biopsy equipment looked like a small gun, like the one they use for piercing your ears. I could see the radiologist trying to find the best place to biopsy the lump. He pressed the tip of the "gun" to my breast and then I heard it go "bang"; one sample was done. Then he sampled a lymph node in another spot, just in case. Bang, it shot off again. I wanted to jump from the noise alone, only I knew it would interfere with the biopsy if I moved. It didn't hurt a lot because of the freezing; there was just a feeling of pressure. After the biopsy was completed, the technician put a thick pressure dressing on the wound and gave me a list of follow-up instructions. She told me not to be afraid if I had a little bleeding from my nipple over the next few days. I left with a huge package of information on breast cancer, and they said that there would be more in the mail.

I tried calling Kevin to pick me up, but he was outside doing some work with my nephew and left the kids to answer the phone. Needless to say, the kids didn't answer the phone. I felt frustrated, stranded and very scared. Then

I remembered my nephew's cell-phone number and called him. Mike answered right away, and Kevin came for me. It was the same day that our beautiful new sunroom was completed.

It is hard to believe that I had an abnormal mammogram, ultrasound and biopsy all in one day. Not only did I have breast cancer, but it was locally *advanced* breast cancer. I felt terribly upset that the cancer had been growing, probably for the whole eight months that I was being treated for mastitis. I felt emotionally and physically stunned. My first thought lying on the examination table was that I was dying, so I wouldn't be tired much longer. I was already feeling as if the life was being "sucked out of me" for at least a month. The power of the unconscious to use metaphor to send us a message is amazing.

I cried when Kevin picked me up, and I told him what had happened. He was initially stunned when he heard the news and then felt terrible that I was not able to reach him by phone. When we got home from the hospital, I called the surgeon's office to tell them that I "flunked" the mammogram, ultrasound and most likely the biopsy all in a single day. I wanted them to know what had happened before my appointment, which was scheduled five days later on the Tuesday September 2, 2008, the day after the Canadian Labour Day holiday weekend.

Later that evening, I really felt like the world was ending. It felt like God had deserted me. I wondered if I would be alive at Christmas. I was terrified that I would die prematurely, just like my mother. History was going to repeat itself! I was going to leave my two children, Eliza and Leonie, alone, just like what had happened to me. I was completely overwhelmed.

Eliza and Leonie knew something was wrong because I was tearful (and probably looked very stressed). Kevin and I talked for a couple of days before telling the girls. Even telling our children was harder than normal because the mother of one of Leonie's best friends was in the hospital dying from a brain tumour. Leonie was very upset and crying with my news. She immediately thought I was going to die. So did I, but I couldn't say those thoughts out loud. Eliza automatically said that I would be fine. She never really allowed herself to think about my death from cancer. Instead, she focused on grade eight, and all her fears and anxieties were projected onto peers, teachers, sports and school work. Both girls wanted to be around me all the time.

Every summer, my brother and sisters and their families come together for a barbeque. This year, the barbeque was planned for the upcoming weekend (Labour Day) to inaugurate our new sunroom. I didn't want to tell my siblings about the cancer that day because I didn't want anybody remembering the party as the last one before I died. I asked Kevin and the girls not to tell my brother and sisters so I could tell them the news after the surgeon's appointment.

Sunday morning we chose to go to Kate's church (an Anglican priest we know) because I wanted to be in a small church where I thought I would feel safer. When I was getting dressed, I noticed blood coming from my right nipple (just like the radiology staff had warned me). I started to cry and put tissue in my bra. I took a sedative when I came home because I wanted to be calm for the party. Everyone seemed to have a good time, even though Kevin, Eliza, Leonie and I were quieter than usual. My siblings left without knowing that I had cancer. I could hardly wait for the party to be over so that I could take off some of the brave face I had assumed.

On the following Tuesday, Eliza and Leonie returned to school after their summer vacation. It was a rather dismal morning. The girls were not excited to meet their new teachers or to see their friends. As we were leaving for the early morning surgeon's appointment, I felt like I was abandoning my daughters on an important day because Kevin and I were not able to be home to see them off before school.

I was lucky that my appointment with Dr. Holiday (my surgeon) was prescheduled because I knew there was no time to waste before treatment needed to begin. I was surprised when Dr. Holiday met me in the patient lobby of the surgical clinic. I figured this was a bad sign. Dr. Holiday and his nurse practitioner, Pat, were very comforting. He told me I had locally advanced breast cancer: "If it looks like a duck, walks like a duck, it is probably a duck." He told me the cancer was very treatable and they had a special treatment protocol for people like me; it would just be a very difficult time for eight to ten months. First you have chemotherapy to shrink the tumour, then surgery and then radiation. He had told me he had a patient just like me in January, and that she did not have any signs of cancer during the surgery after chemo and that she had reconstructive surgery only the past Friday. I was surprised when he told me that he had already gone to the radiology department at the breast screening clinic and looked at my mammogram and ultrasound from January and February, 2008 and August 28th. (It made me feel like he was a very thorough doctor and it increased my feelings of safety under his care.) He said he could not see any signs of cancer in February. He then explained I would be scheduled for the diagnostic tests (MRI, CT scan and bone scan) over the next week to determine the extent of the cancer. Dr. Holiday said he would contact an oncologist who specialized in locally advanced breast cancer. According to the protocol, I would be seen in the next week or so. I have included a table of all of the dates to better describe the whirlwind of appointments that took place in just over one week.

The MRI was scheduled for the next day. Lesley, one of my best friends, came with me to the appointment. Lesley was a good choice to accompany me because she is a registered nurse and her cousin was a ten-year survivor of breast cancer. I was so nervous, and Lesley was so calming because of her grounded personality.

During the MRI, I was asked to lie down on a table with my breasts hanging in a contraption; then my body was placed in the MRI machine. The technicians gave me ear plugs to lessen the clicking noise of the MRI machine. It was too bad the ear plugs couldn't reduce the banging sound of my beating heart. The sedative that I took prior to the appointment really helped. One test was behind me.

Chronology of Medical Appointments and Family Activities:
August 28, 2008 to September 16, 2008

Sunday	Monday	Tuesday	Wednesday	Thursday	Friday	Saturday
				Aug. 28 - Breast Screening Mammogram, Ultrasound, Biopsy		
Aug. 31 - Family Picnic		Sept. 1 - First Day of School 8:30 Dr. Holiday Surgeon	Sept. 2 - MRI			
Sept. 6 - Kevin to Victoria, B.C. Eliza and Leonie to a sleepover	Sept. 7 - 7:00 CT scan of chest and abdomen	Sept. 8 - Results of MRI Decision for double mastectomy	Sept. 9 - Results of CT scan.	Sept. 10 - 8:30 injection of isotope for bone scan 10:00 mammogram 11:30 actual bone scan	Sept. 11- Results of Bone Scan	

August 28, 2008 to September 16, 2008 - continued						
Sunday	Monday	Tuesday	Wednesday	Thursday	Friday	Saturday
Sept. 14 - Kevin returns from Victoria Potvin	Sept. 15 - Our anniversary. 9:00 Meeting with Dr. Potvin oncologist.	Sept. 16 - First Day of Chemo				

Unfortunately, Kevin had to leave for Victoria, BC, that weekend, for a week, so I was alone with the girls for my remaining diagnostic tests. Life felt like a rollercoaster that was hurtling out of control. Even though the girls had already seen me crying and knew I had breast cancer, they were really upset when they found out they would have to sleep over at their friends' houses on Sunday night because my appointment for the CT scan was Monday at 7:00 a.m. The girls cried as they left for their friends on Sunday evening. Neither one of them wanted to go, but there wasn't a choice.

Over the weekend, I started becoming progressively more afraid of having the CT scan because I feared I would have an allergic reaction to the dye that they would be injecting. Lesley knew about my phobia about anaphylaxis (a serious allergic reaction to a substance) that I have carried since I was about twenty years old (i.e. for thirty years), so she took another day off of work to go with me to the CT scan to support me. (That is a really a sign of a good friend,) In the radiology department, I mentioned to Lesley how nice it was for the staff to bring me some water to drink. Lesley laughed because I hadn't realized the "water" was actually an oral contrast material they use for the CT scan (to make the bowel show up more clearly on the test). For the first time, I realized I had already been given both an oral contrast material and intravenous dye in the fall of 2007 and had been needlessly anxious about having an anaphylactic reaction. The technician took me into the CT scan machine and injected the dye intravenously, saying, "It's going to make your bladder feel warm," and it did. I made it through that test as well. I decided that from this day forward I would consider having a phobia of anaphylaxis as a "luxury" item, especially given the chemotherapy that I would be receiving.

The following day, Pat (Dr. Holiday's nurse practitioner) called to tell me the MRI results showed there was "something" in my other breast as well. The doctors wanted me to go for a mammogram of my left breast later that week. Now I was really hysterical. I was so frightened that this meant the cancer had already spread throughout my whole body. I decided right there and then to have a double mastectomy. I never again wanted to repeat the stress of mammograms. Mammograms are often considered the gold standard test for finding breast cancer. They were certainly not sensitive to breast cancer in my case; I would never be able to trust the results in the future. I mentioned that I was having the bone scan on Thursday, so they asked me to be injected with the isotope for the bone scan in the morning (8:30 a.m.) and then to come directly over for the mammogram.

On Wednesday, Pat, Dr. Holiday's nurse practitioner, called and said the CT scan of my abdomen and chest was normal. I felt so relieved to hear this news. I also felt comforted when she told me that MRIs are often oversensitive and can find things that are actually normal. The biopsy results identified the cancer in my right breast as slow growing and very sensitive to estrogen. She told me she would call and tell me the results of Thursday's bone scan the next day. I never knew doctors could get test results so quickly. Pat said they make exceptions in important cases.

Lesley once again took another day off to take me to my appointments on Thursday. After the mammogram, the technician told me the mass that was seen on the MRI in my left breast was a cyst. I started to laugh because it was the only possible reaction I could have. I said, "Forgive me for laughing, but I was told the same thing for the right breast for years and now I have advanced breast cancer." I said I was going to have a double mastectomy and I would never have another mammogram again.

On Friday afternoon, I found out from Pat the bone scan was negative! I was elated at the end of a very stressful week of tests and waiting for the results. It was comforting to know there were no other measurable masses outside of the breast; no one had felt any lumps in my armpit or neck. I knew that this news did not rule out microscopic cancerous cells in the rest of my body, but I felt a surge of hope that I would survive the cancer. Pat told me my first oncologist appointment was the following Monday, September 15th.

Eliza and Leonie continued to be upset throughout the week, and Kevin was still away half a continent away in Victoria. I gave the girls as much support as I was able, but I knew that what I could offer was not enough. On

Thursday, September 11th, I was so tired I called Mary Poppins[2] (my friend of twenty-five years and the girls' godmother) to come to our house and spend the night on Friday. The girls were originally supposed to go to her house, but they did not feel they could leave me. Mary Poppins changed her plans and came to stay with us. I made dinner and went to bed early. As I fell asleep, I heard them laughing and having a good time. Mary Poppins spent the night, and on Saturday morning we went shopping to a knitting store. We both made purchases. I was going to make a cotton afghan for my new sunroom in order to keep my mind off of the cancer. Even though I was very tired after shopping, I drove Mary Poppins home. In retrospect, I wish I had asked her husband Ken (Mr. Poppins) to pick her up and relieve me of the drive.

There was a terrible rain storm in London, Ontario, on Sunday night when Kevin was flying back from Victoria, BC. The wind was so strong it blew part of the eavestrough off of the new sunroom. I was really worried that Kevin's flight would be cancelled by the storm and that he would not be back in time for my oncology appointment the next morning. I waited up until midnight when Kevin finally arrived home. Once again we had to leave early for my first appointment with my oncologist, Dr. Potvin, so Eliza and Leonie had to leave for school on their own.

Monday, September 15th was my eighteenth wedding anniversary, and Dr. Potvin gave me the best present anyone could offer. She explained that even though I had locally advanced breast cancer, she would *cure* me (even though it would be a rotten year because of the treatment). The good news was the tumour was sensitive to estrogen, but further tests would be needed to identify whether the tumour was sensitive to the "HER" protein treatment (another biological marker to tell the type of cancer). Dr. Potvin examined the tumour in my right breast and measured it with her hand. It was now the size of a cantaloupe. She told me it was a good thing that the tumour was not attached to the chest wall, which would lead to a better outcome from the surgical perspective. She explained the chemotherapy to me: I would receive intravenous (IV) chemo every three weeks. First, I would have one set of four doses of two IV drugs, and then I would have four doses of another drug. I would also take a high dose of a steroid drug to prevent a serious reaction to the chemo. Each Friday before my chemo, I would have blood work completed to ensure my white blood count was high enough to proceed; I would be weighed because the steroid drug often caused women to gain weight, which was upsetting news since I was already overweight; and my oncology team would review my progress and answer any questions. During the appointment, I would meet with at least one member of Dr. Potvin's health care team, consisting of Dr. B., a general practitioner, Lynn, a nurse practitioner, and Mary Anne, a registered nurse.

The first four treatments would be one and a half hours long every three weeks. After chemo, I would be nauseous for about three days. She said that 80 percent of people are fine on chemo, but 20 percent of people will have trouble metabolizing the drugs. Dr. Potvin said the chemo works for about ten days, and then the body heals for the next ten days; however, the body never gets a chance to completely heal before the next treatment. One of the most serious side effects would be the drop in my white blood cells (the cells that fight infection). She was emphatic that if my temperature went up to 38° C (37° C is considered normal), it was a medical emergency related to infection and depressed white blood cells and that I needed to come to the hospital right away for intravenous antibiotics or they may not be able to save me from the infection. I would probably lose my hair after the second treatment. Dr. Potvin advised me not to work through this period; however, I explained how important my work was to me. Work has always been such an important part of my identity; I wanted to feel like I could contribute through my research. I promised I would only work if I was able. Dr. Potvin said the chemotherapy would begin the next day. I was surprised that she spent almost forty-five minutes with me and was attentive the whole time. It once again made me feel like I was safe under her care.

I read in some of the breast cancer literature that children sometimes react negatively to the baldness that comes with chemotherapy and that wigs can provide a sense of normalcy. After the meeting with Dr. Potvin, Kevin and I went shopping to buy a wig. To my surprise the salesperson told us a synthetic wig would melt near a hot stove. I have never been naturally domestic and I immediately envisioned melting the wig the first day I wore it. I left the store a new owner of a human hair wig.

By that evening, I was more affirmed in my decision to make myself live for Kevin and the girls. I tried to think about my anniversary as marking the choice to live. We went out to dinner as a family to one of our favourite Italian restaurants. I had a couple of beers. It was going to be my last chemo-free time for about six months, and I wanted to remember the night. It was a good night. In some ways it felt like it was my "Last Supper" before treatment.

I started chemotherapy the next day, September 16, 2008. I would have just been having the biopsy now if I had decided to postpone the biopsy for three weeks (the next available appointment). Clearly, it was life-saving decision when I made the choice to have the biopsy on August 28th, rather than waiting. It was also a life-saving decision to accept chemotherapy, some of the most potent drugs available (poison to cancer cells and poison to many healthy cells). I never felt I had a choice on whether or not I would accept the chemotherapy because I knew I needed to try everything to live for my girls; the sooner chemo could begin, the sooner it could fight the cancer. Clearly my body wasn't able to fight the cancer alone.

I had telephoned my family the previous week to tell them I had breast cancer. I can't remember how they reacted, but I think they were shocked. Next, I told Charlene, my supervisor at work, who was great and agreed to allow me to work from home, as I was able. Fortunately I was a researcher and didn't have to work in an office. I never would have been able to continue working if I still held a management position that required me to supervise staff and attend meetings most of the day.

The next step was to tell other people about my cancer. I found the process re-traumatizing each time I repeated the message. I was so upset at the idea of telling anyone else because I worried people might write me off or feel sorry for me. To my surprise, it was a humbling experience telling people, but not for the reasons I had previously thought. I discovered that many people remembered things I had done to help them. People I hardly knew were praying for me and wishing me well. Such surprising affirmations were comforting and encouraged me to face the treatment. I told everyone I would keep them up to date on my progress between treatments.

Many people who have had cancer talk about beginning a pronounced period of self-reflection, and I was no different. I realized I have wanted people to care about me throughout my whole life. I realized I have genuinely cared about people, but I often hoped that people would care for me in return. I suffered many tragic losses as a child. My father left my childhood family when I was a year old, and my mother died when I was five years old. Even though my grandpa raised me and my four siblings for another five years, he died when I was ten years old. In order to keep me and my siblings together, we were placed under the care of housekeepers who were not really interested in our emotional well being. I was ignored and neglected. I had been self-aware for a long time, and my early life became the default position in defining the rest of my life. I knew my frequent feelings of abandonment and inadequacy were usually generated from my childhood. I knew I harboured anger and resentment from these childhood experiences. As an adult, I believe I desperately tried to put these feelings behind me, rather than dealing with them. Now I realized I had to face the anger, fear of abandonment and resentment because these memories took up way too much energy that was needed for healing. I knew I needed to re-evaluate my life over the next few weeks and really examine what was important to me.

Reflections:

- Everyone is relieved to hear they don't have cancer. In my case it was a false hope. I wish I had asked for a biopsy when the lump did not go away.
- Sometimes people say that cancer is painless. Mine was always painful.

- Health-care professionals may rule out cancer when they hear the results from a radiologist. In my case, appointments were delayed because the mammogram and ultrasound were negative six months earlier.
- I wish I had listened more to my body when it was so tired. I wish I had paid more attention to the message, "I feel like my life is being sucked out of me."
- Neoplasm sounds much nicer than cancer, but a prettier-sounding word does not make it less dangerous.
- I wondered if it would be difficult to trust the health-care system again when I felt it let me down. In the future, I wondered if "normal" results would comfort me or would I continue to worry that there were just undetected problems?
- I was very fortunate with my health care team right away. I felt I could trust them immediately. My team was very supportive when the breast cancer was identified. Dr. Potvin's words "I can cure you; it is just going to be a difficult year" resonated with me and gave me some desperately needed hope. Whenever I felt like I was dying, I would remember her words of hope over and over.
- Waiting for pre-chemo results is very anxiety producing. Perhaps I should have had more faith, but I couldn't find the energy.
- It is almost impossible to absorb all of the information that is given to you.
- Surviving past trauma reminded me that I have survived terrible things before.
- While I mentioned I was worried about cancer to Kevin and my close friends, I never mentioned these fears to my young daughters, Eliza and Leonie, before my diagnosis.

- It is really hard to tell your children. We all worried and became stressed in our own ways.
- Kevin and the girls were the biggest motivators to make me want to live.
- Friends who take you to appointments and listen to you are invaluable supports.
- Telling people about my cancer was traumatizing. There were a lot of tears.
- It was traumatizing for me to hear people's stories about individuals who valiantly fought cancer and tragically died. I began to ask people to only tell me the story if there was a happy ending. I did not need to add anything to my arsenal of fear.
- Family and friends may not be able to cope with the news and provide the support you really need.
- Praying didn't relieve my fears. I just hoped that God was listening.

Invincible
Eliza, Age Fourteen

August 28, 2008, is the day that will torment my heart forever. The day that I wished I was an emotionless zombie bound to walk the earth for eternity. The day I found out the truth about the thin line between life and death. I fear to say these words aloud, for if they are not spoken, I can believe they don't exist and life can continue to spin as innocent as ever. But these words are the truth, and I must learn to live in the reality that no one is invincible, not even the one person who promised to be there no matter what.

August 28, 2008, is the day that my mother was diagnosed with advanced breast cancer. The day that the world stopped being innocent and became the unforgiving world it is today.

I wish I could say that this event was easy to overcome, but unfortunately that would be a lie. It feels as if this event will always eat at my heart till there is nothing left but an empty space. The knowledge and fear from this experience still haunts my every waking moment. Sometimes I still fear to get out of bed. I now look upon faces that I know and love hoping that I will have a chance to see them again.

My mother is a survivor of cancer. From this experience, I now realize that you should tell everyone how much you love them and live every day to the fullest because it could be your last.

Chapter 2

Good Friday: Chemotherapy

Jesus' passion is something I thought a great deal about during my treatment. He suffered during the trial, carrying the cross and finally on the cross. His body was pierced with nails and a sword. He was humbled publicly. The biggest difference between Jesus and me was that he suffered willingly to save others. Not me! I didn't want to die. I wanted to live for my children. I travelled through Good Friday never feeling treatment was a choice. Even though many people repeatedly told me how courageous I was, in reality I always knew I was a coward.

I think chemotherapy was a bit akin to the time after Jesus was arrested in the garden. There were moments of physical pain and discomfort, but it wasn't every moment. It was mainly the fear of what would happen next. Travelling back and forth between clinics and doctors' appointments, I wondered when I would meet Pontius Pilate who would pronounce a death sentence.

This next section often emphasizes the physical suffering. You just can't get away from its reality during treatment. The emotional and spiritual sufferings co-exist, but the story of physical suffering must be told first. Sometimes the ashes of suffering need to be scraped away to enable us to hear the meaning of the emotional and spiritual suffering.

Chemo Time

Chemo time feels like a time zone very similar to Eastern Standard, Central, Mountain and Pacific Standard Time, but the closest analogy, though, is Daylight Savings Time as the clock springs forward. During this transition, you end up feeling mixed up and wondering where the missing time went. For the first few days, everything feels out of kilter; then you start to adjust. This is what happens during chemo time. Your whole world starts to shift around the events of the three-week cycles of chemo. How many days to the next chemo? When do I start my steroid drugs? When will the side effects start to appear? How many days does the chemo work? Will it work? Will the tumour shrink? Then all of a sudden you become focused on healing before the next dose. There is nothing more frightening than thinking your chemo will be delayed because of an infection or your white blood cell count is too low. It is especially nerve wracking when you feel and see the tumour in your breast every day reminding you of your mortality. Could eight doses of chemo really make a difference to saving my life?

Everyone responds to chemo differently, but I think we are all hoping for a miracle. Prior to my first chemo, I began to prepare myself psychologically. I mentally and emotionally invited the chemo to work by thinking of it like communion in church. Most of all, my experience with cancer has been a very spiritual experience because I felt I needed more than the world of medicine to survive this cancer. I followed Kate's advice to use a spiritual image during my chemo to comfort me. Therefore before and during my chemo, I would recite multiple times "the Lord is my Shepherd" and the communion hymn "Eat this bread, drink this cup, come to me and never be hungry. Eat this bread, drink this cup, trust in me and you will not thirst."[3] I then found it comforting to put in my personal petitions to God such as never be lonely, never be sick etc. In the past, I often had a feeling of doom and the need for personal sacrifice when reciting "Thy will be done" in the Lord's Prayer. All at once, I discovered in church that listening to the Lord's Prayer being sung "warmed" this sentence for me, and it began to become a source of comfort, even though it did not reduce my worries for the future.

Dr. Bernie Siegel[4] is considered a cancer "guru" by many, so when Kate gave me a copy of one of his books, I took her suggestion and read it. He talked of cancer "super star" survivors, but this message did not inspire me; in fact it had the opposite effect. I thought the cancer "super stars" were all exceptional, and I recoiled thinking there was absolutely no way I could be a "super star." There is a strong possibility that I misinterpreted the book, but I had difficulty engaging in Dr. Siegel's visualization exercises to help get rid of the cancer and cope through treatment. I failed the first few tests. I couldn't get beyond feeling the cancer was similar to a blocked milk duct, even though the tumour was now the size of a cantaloupe. I couldn't visualize killing the cancer with chemo because I knew the cancer was part of my body and somehow I had created it. I was able to visualize the chemo going to the cancer cells and telling them they were no longer needed. I wanted the cancer cells to feel warm and relaxed in order to let the chemo come in so the cancer cells could realize it was time to leave. This was totally anthropomorphism.

Dr. Siegel also suggested that a person should try to visualize him or herself living to be ninety years old. I found this impossible, so I made a joke of it. Nancy, one of the administrative assistants at work, designed a picture of me at age 90 according to my description of myself with large muscles and with my grandchildren. I had talked with Nancy about wanting to live long enough to have grandchildren, so she used a picture I had never seen of Eliza and Leonie at a picnic to represent my future grandchildren. It was comforting to assume my future grandchildren would actually look like my children now. I also started a contest at work to choose the best wig and received many humorous pictures that helped relieve the tensions of the day.

Like Joseph, in the Old Testament, I reflected on dreams to help me understand my feelings and surmise if there were any important messages to comfort or help me. The night before my first chemo treatment, I dreamt I was tied up in a gypsy caravan wagon. There was a venomous snake in a cage beside me, and people were going to stick it on my neck right on the jugular vein. When they opened the cage, I was full of panic, but to my surprise, a beautiful, sleek white cat jumped out. The cat jumped on my lap and purred for a few minutes, then casually jumped off and left. The white cat in this dream symbolized safety and really reassured me that, maybe, I would not be in danger from the chemo. The chemo would help me.

Even though I am a registered nurse, I chose not to remember most of the names of the chemotherapy drugs and especially didn't want to hear about the negative side effects of these drugs. I was convinced I would experience anticipatory worrying and imagine that every possible side effect would happen to me. Therefore, I decided to focus on preventing the biggest threat, which was "infection," rather than focusing on the individual side effects of the chemo drugs. The nurses told me I could call the nursing telephone help (triage) line if I had questions, and that is exactly what I opted to do. I knew I was strong and healthy from working out with weights, walking and riding a stationary bike prior to September. Given I was already the "queen" of contingency planning, I was amazed that for the first time in my life I decided to wait and see what happened before trying to deal with it.

Someone suggested to me that I should identify an inner support group with whom I would like to share my worries and concerns. I chose Karen, my childhood friend of over forty years, Lesley, a registered nurse and friend for twenty years, Elaine, another long-term friend of twenty years who lives in Victoria, BC, and Kate, an Anglican priest with whom I have had dinner parties for about four years. I am very fortunate to know such caring and capable people. They were the ones to whom I told my innermost fears.

Chemo #1

On my first day of chemo (September 16th), I knew I was not physically well. I felt exhausted most of the time (afternoon naps and being in bed by 8:30 p.m.), and I had a constant pain in my right breast and shoulder. I was very anxious and feeling overwhelmed on the morning of the first chemo treatment. I took a sedative so I would not start crying in the clinic. When I had asked Dr. Potvin if it would be okay to take the sedative, she said it would be fine and it could even reduce the anticipatory nausea. The sedative worked, and I did not begin crying or embarrassing myself during the treatment, which was a great relief to me.

The cancer clinic is a very open space where all patients and their families wait. On checking in for the appointment, the receptionist gave me a beeper so Kevin and I could walk around if we wanted before I was summoned. The beeper was on vibration mode, and I jumped as the beeper vibrated in my hand. Kevin and I entered the chemo room together because one family member is allowed to stay with the patient throughout the treatment. The chemo room was very large and had at least fifty spots for people in two open rooms, but only one room had windows. The chemo nurse was wonderful. She welcomed me, and then she started the IV. She explained the drugs. First you get the antiemetic and steroid through the IV, then the red drug. I heard another patient called it the "red devil" later in my treatment, and by then I knew why. The red devil really attacks both cancerous and normal cells. There was also another drug, but I didn't want to know about it. I only asked for the side effects that I needed to report to them. I kept repeating to myself (almost like a chant) that everyone responds individually. I didn't want to become too anxious and worry myself into having the side effects. The chemo session went fine. I even had the energy to visit the wig shop again on the way home from the appointment.

At supper I felt hungry. Kevin made meatballs, and they smelled good. Right after I ate, I knew it was a mistake because almost immediately I got indigestion with severe burning in my stomach that lasted throughout the week. I was able to handle the nausea the first evening, but at 2:00 a.m. I was awake, emotionally agitated and experiencing pain from indigestion. I took the anti-nausea medication, and one of the side effects was that I became even more wired. I didn't know it at the time, but the steroid drug can make a person very excitable (almost manic) and unable to sleep. That night in my restlessness, I had an ongoing dream. It was like my body was scanning for cancer cells. I would slightly arouse and think "lungs clear." I'd go back to sleep and arouse, "abdomen clear." Next my bones were clear. I awoke in the morning thinking maybe I would be okay. My subconscious was trying to tell me the chemo was working.

The gastric pain continued, and it especially hurt when I ate. Four days later I was in terrible gastric pain and my abdomen was very swollen. I called the triage line at the cancer clinic, and they ordered a drug to reduce the acid in the stomach. Unfortunately, I didn't know I needed to call the pharmacy to find out if it was ready. I went another day in terrible pain before I realized that the drug may already be at the pharmacy. Kevin picked up the drug, and I took it right away. By that evening, the pain was so severe I thought I was dying. My abdomen was so bloated. I took a shower because I did not want to die knowing my body wasn't freshly showered. (Interesting the thoughts we have.) I asked Kevin to lie beside me and hold my hand. I didn't want to leave home. I finally fell asleep. That was the worst night of my chemo. The next morning, I felt a bit better because I could tell the stomach medicine was beginning to work. While I was sick, Leonie also had a gastric illness. I do not know if I also had a stomach virus in addition to the effects of the steroid drug. I do know it was a terrible experience for six days after the first dose of chemo and then the side effects passed.

After the weekend, I told Kate (my friend, the Anglican priest) about my terrible experience thinking that I was dying. She listened to my fears and witnessed my tears. Her advice was to try and understand my fears instead of running from them. She told me that you are never alone in feeling fear. It is one of the most common experiences of life shared by many other people. She suggested that I read *The Places That Scare You*[5] (a book written by a Buddhist nun) and *The Gift of Courage*[6], and they were very helpful. Kate didn't say it, but I imagine Jesus had to have been afraid of dying at some point.

Eliza and Leonie were worried about me during this first treatment. Leonie continued to cry and have headaches and stomach aches every day since she heard about the diagnosis. She was so stressed that a big clump of her hair fell out, and she had a bald spot on her head about seven centimeters in diameter. Leonie was also struggling with her worries about her friend whose mother was in the hospital dying of cancer in addition to her desperate fear that her own mother could also be dying of cancer. She missed weeks of school because she felt physically and emotionally unwell. In contrast, Eliza projected all of her worries somewhere else. She focused on the social politics of grade eight and making the volleyball team. Kevin was busy trying to do all of the errands (groceries, etc.) and trying to support the whole family, but it was just too overwhelming with my neediness and his demanding job. Luckily, Kevin's career is flexible and he was able to come with me to all of my doctor's appointments and chemo treatments, which I found invaluable since my memory was not as sound as usual related to the stress. Kevin took notes, writing down the information received at every visit so we could talk about how the appointment went later in the evening.

At the end of September, Kevin, Eliza and Leonie went to the cancer clinic for a family support night. The parent's session was separate from the children's. The cancer clinic offered some exercises around coping during treatment, and the girls saw where I was receiving my chemo treatment and where I would have radiation. It was a good information session, but I knew they would need much more than informational support.

Kevin and I continued to go to Kate's church because it was such a comfortable group. The Church of the Hosannas is a small congregation (about twenty people). Kevin and I could sit at the back of the church by ourselves so I didn't have to worry about any physical contact that could lead to infection. I did not share the sign of peace with people, and they were very understanding. Because I was raised in the United Church of Canada and we were very unfamiliar with the liturgy of the Anglican Church, Kate gave me a book so I could read some of the liturgy. I found having weekly communion very comforting, and it helped me feel like I could heal. We decided to stay at Hosannas so I could have weekly communion (our United Church only has communion about five times at year).

In terms of employment, it was very fortunate that I was employed as a nurse researcher/educator at the local health unit. My director, Charlene, my research assistant, Ashley, and Gayle in human resources were incredibly supportive. Charlene agreed to allow me to work at home as I was able, and she even arranged for me to be set up at home with wireless internet. This meant a great deal to me. In August, I had been fortunate to obtain a research grant, and I really wanted to follow the research process to the end. I also had some journal manuscripts I wanted to publish. I know some people may think that I was crazy for trying to work during this stressful period, but my normal work routine helped to keep my mind occupied, preventing me from thinking about my possible death.

One of the least-known side effects of chemo and working at home is the need to renovate your surroundings. Our new sunroom floor was lovely, but it made the rest of the house look rather shabby. So we decided to replace the old floor in the kitchen, hallway and entrance way with the same flooring that was in the sunroom. We also put in a water-efficient toilet and started construction on the new deck. My nephew Mike completed the work during the first few days after chemo. With Mike present, I was not afraid of being alone and needing help, and we also had many opportunities for one-on-one discussion.

On the tenth day after chemo, I experienced a positive effect from the chemo, but I did not know it right away. All at once I felt this warmth in my breast. I felt a little panicky and thought, *Oh, now what?* The warmth shot up to my armpit, and in one big swoosh, the swelling in my breast disappeared. I couldn't believe it after just one chemo treatment. It had to be working!

I started losing my hair on the thirteenth day. My doctors and nurses mentioned it would happen between two to three weeks. When my hair started to fall out, it came out in huge clumps. Eliza couldn't believe her eyes and was in a frenzy pulling it out. It was like gallows humour, and we were both laughing as my hair fell out as if it was never attached in the first place. The next day I called my hairdresser, Farzaneh, and she gave me a buzz cut. I brought my wig to the appointment, and she trimmed it a bit so it would look like my regular hairstyle. There was only one problem: after I lost my hair, I was unable to turn my head without the wig moving in a different direction. I only ended up wearing the wig one day to show Kevin and his coworkers, and then I put it away and wore toques. Over the next few days, my hair fell out completely when I was washing it with a washcloth in the shower. I must admit that this time it bothered me to watch the last of my hair fall out and see it go down the shower drain. Because I had never believed myself to be physically attractive in the past, my lack of hair didn't affect my self-image too much after those first few days.

Chemotherapy makes you really think about your lifestyle, and I was determined to start taking better care of myself, thinking if I ate better, slept enough and exercised, things would go better for me. I used to walk around four km a day, so I adapted by walking around the block so I didn't get too far away from home in case I didn't feel well and needed to get back in a hurry. (My block is 0.8 km in circumference.) I rode the stationary exercise bike and lifted my weights (mind you, I decreased the amount of weight I was lifting). Not a drop of alcohol passed my lips after the first chemo treatment. Certainly the gastric problems had a lot to do with the decision not to drink alcohol. I was still very tired every day, and I took a daily afternoon nap for about an hour and was in bed for the night by 8:30 p.m. During my afternoon nap, I put the electric blanket on at about the same temperature as the clothes dryer. It was hot under the blankets. Lance Armstrong, the famous bicycle rider who had testicular cancer, talked about heating up the body by riding his racing bike. My thinking was that if I heated my body up enough then the chemo could better circulate to all of the areas where the cancer lay hidden. I don't know if any of this was magical thinking, but each nap made me feel like I was actively doing something to get better. That thought alone helped me get through the day.

There were many nights I was restless during my treatment and I would go down to the sunroom and sit in the dark and pray. I would mainly pray for others because I have never been good at praying for myself. I think that being a nurse has helped me in my ability to pray for people. I would visualize people's bodies healing and pray for it to happen. One day I mentioned to Kate I was so tired that all I could do was pray. She looked me straight in the eye and asked me why I thought that praying didn't count as work.

Every third weekend during my chemo, my friend Karen came to visit and Kevin took the girls to see his mother so I could get more rest. Eliza and Leonie usually wanted to be around me every minute, and I think the reason for this behaviour was two-fold. First, the girls were comforted by talking to me about their lives, and second, I think they thought they could protect me if they were with me. However, I needed some time alone and time with my friend so that I would not always feel on call.

I am very fortunate to have Karen as my friend. Being around Karen gave me hope that I could survive the cancer because for the past forty years, she has seen me survive so many crises. We could talk about things that concerned us in life and not just cancer. I understood early that it is a terrible feeling to have cancer as your master identity rather than mother, wife, researcher, etc. Karen was studying for her PhD, and when we were together, we would talk about her courses. This gave me a sense of purpose, that I could still help someone else. For a few hours, I was a friend, confidante and helper. I still felt tired after these weekends, but I always felt better having Karen present.

At the end of the first three-week cycle of chemo, I went for my follow-up appointment at the cancer clinic. Lynn, the nurse practitioner, went over the information about the cancer again and answered my questions. I discovered I had retained very little of the information from the first visit. I told Lynn I had recovered pretty well from the first chemo and was grateful for the chance to heal. My tumour now measured 17.5 cm by 17.5 cm, the size of a very large navel orange, but much smaller than a cantaloupe. Since the first chemo, I had visualized my white blood cell count (WBC) as recovering quickly and being high enough to continue with the second treatment of chemo. If the WBC count is less than 1.3, the chemo is postponed. It was such a terrible shock to me when I came for my pre-chemo appointment only to discover that my WBCs were only 0.7 x 109/litre. Lynn told me about a special drug that would increase my WBCs. The drug had to be administered subcutaneously (a needle under the skin). The most shocking part was the drug cost over $2,600 per dose and I would need seven doses. There was no way we could afford to pay over $18,000. Fortunately, my benefit plan covered the drug, which was a huge relief because I was convinced it would help save my life. Instead of postponing my second chemo treatment, the treatment team decided to retest my WBCs in three days, the same day as my next scheduled chemo. It was a depressing weekend because I had visualized a better outcome and these efforts failed to get the result I wanted: enough white blood cells. Fortunately, my WBC count was 1.3 on Monday, and the second chemo could proceed as scheduled.

Chemo #2

Before I discuss the second chemo, I want to provide some background information about Leonie. Kevin and I very much wanted a second child, but instead I had five very depressing and traumatic miscarriages. After my fifth emergency surgery because of another miscarriage, we decided to adopt. Since Eliza wanted a baby sister, we decided to adopt a baby girl. We chose international adoption because we thought we were more likely be successful at adopting the first time, as compared to a domestic adoption. We chose Guatemala because Kevin has Spanish heritage and he and Eliza have Spanish colouring. The adoption process took two years before Kevin, Eliza, and I were able to travel to Guatemala and bring Leonie home as our daughter when she was two years old. Leonie fell in love with Kevin at first site in Guatemala, but I still think she was traumatized from leaving her foster family because sometimes she would awake in the middle of the night with "night screams" and we couldn't touch her until she recognized who we were. I am providing this information because Leonie continued to really struggle with my diagnosis. I believe she may have experienced latent separation anxiety because a two-year-old child would probably have a physical memory of the separation from her foster family. From September onward, Leonie cried every day and had stomach aches. She missed school at least half of the time. Leonie knew she was upset, but she could never verbally pinpoint her feelings. Leonie would cry and say she hurt inside and was upset, but she was unable to articulate why she was upset and could not cope with her emotions and physical aches and pains. Leonie was old enough to know that I could die but too young to really understand the relationship between her fears and her emotional and physical wellbeing. In addition, Leonie was facing the fact that the mom of one of her best friends had just died at the end of September. I wondered if the death of her friend's mom and my life-threatening illness reawakened some old memories of separation anxiety.

When Leonie was two years old, she caught scarlet fever from a strep infection, and subsequently had many strep infections afterwards. The night before my second chemo, Leonie complained of a sore throat. Since strep is contagious and because I was frightened I would get a serious bacterial infection due to my depressed immune system, we isolated Leonie in her room on Sunday night. Leonie was upset because not only was she was feeling sick, she was also feeling isolated. Eliza was also upset because she had to miss a special day planned at school because we needed her to stay home with her sister while we went to chemo. There was no one else available to help us!

Chemo two went fine. I took a sedative about one hour before I left home to calm myself. During the drive to the cancer clinic, I started reciting the Lord's Prayer, the Lord is my Shepherd, and relating the experience of chemo to communion. As I entered the chemo clinic, the routine began. I checked in at reception and was given a beeper; the beeper went off; the nurse greeted me and took me to a chair in the clinic; the IV went in; the IV drugs were administered; the IV came out; I picked up my drugs at the cancer clinic pharmacy, and we went home.

Chemo was a bit more stressful this time, however, because we were worried about Leonie and we wanted to go straight home to see how she was feeling. Kevin took Leonie to our family doctor in the afternoon, just in case she had strep throat, and Dr. Kumar took a throat swab. Leonie was very upset that she was ill and confined to her room which meant that she was not in close proximity to me, especially since Kevin went back to work and Eliza went back to school. I would go to Leonie's door and talk to her without going into her room. I brought her meals to her door just like a prison guard. I felt terrible inside, but I couldn't get over my fear of infection.

The day after chemo I asked Lynn, the mother of one of Leonie's friends, a practising registered nurse, to come over while I gave myself my first needle to build my white blood cells. I was worried about having an allergic reaction (my anaphylaxis phobia didn't disappear overnight). Little did I know that I was so pumped up with steroids it would have been almost impossible to have an allergic reaction. Lynn and I went through the routine of giving a subcutaneous injection: take the medication out of the refrigerator to warm it up; get rid of the bubbles in the needle; look to see if the solution isn't discoloured; pick a site on the abdomen and clean it with the alcohol swab; get ready to inject and then do it. I was perplexed when the needle was supposed to automatically retract, but didn't. It took me a couple of minutes to figure out I was supposed to push a section of the needle over its sharp point. I discarded the needle and then we made friendly chatter while I waited to see if I would react. I survived the injection without any problems, and I was really glad for the extra support!

Leonie continued to be confined to her bedroom until Wednesday morning when I let her come out of her room because she was feeling better, and I assumed the throat swab was negative because we hadn't heard any news from the doctor's office. I figured if the swab was negative, I would no longer be at risk of a strep infection and I started to relax. I felt panicked at 4:30 p.m. when I checked the phone messages only to find out that Dr. Kumar's office had left a message earlier in the day to tell us Leonie did have strep throat. To make matters worse, Leonie had been out of her room and around me most of the day. I rushed to call my doctor's office because they closed at 4:30 pm. Fortunately, Dr. Kumar agreed to phone in a prescription for Leonie's antibiotics to our local pharmacy. It wasn't her policy to give out prescriptions over the phone, but she did it because I was so upset. I then called the cancer clinic to get advice because I was worried about infection. I also called the pharmacist and asked if they could fill the prescription as soon as possible. I felt so vulnerable. Then I waited for the symptoms to strike like a death knell.

On the Friday before Thanksgiving weekend, Kevin complained of a sore throat. I broke down in sobbing tears. I knew I could no longer cope with all of the stress and decided I needed to leave our home and go and stay somewhere safer. I called many friends to see if I could go to their houses, but either they weren't home or it felt to me like there was "no room at the inn." Kate said I could go to her home for a few hours, and I left immediately. At Kate's house I made a few more calls. Luckily, Mr. Poppins answered the phone and said I could come over. I arrived and promptly fell asleep from exhaustion.

The two days I spent at the Poppins were very good for me because I spent much of the time alone, sleeping or reading. I was ill again with the same side effects as the first chemo, but this time the side effects of the chemo didn't seem so bad because I wasn't taking care of the family's needs at the same time. Since I had been sick, the stress in our home exacerbated the fighting between Kevin and Eliza. I knew that this ongoing stress was very unhealthy for me, so I called home and talked to Kevin and Eliza. I explained I could no longer deal with their constant fighting and could not come home until they resolved how they were going to treat each other. I was very direct telling them both they were being selfish: always having to be right, ignoring each other's feelings and ignoring the stress they were causing me with their negative emotions and the constant chaos. Kevin and Eliza each assumed I was siding with the other person. Both agreed to change, and I was relieved to be able to come home that night. For a week, I pointed out each time when they sniped at each other and asked them if they could rephrase what they wanted to say in a more engaging approach. Within a week, the sniping was really reduced; they were treating each other much better and both of them looked more relaxed. I can only imagine how stressful it was for Kevin and Eliza to be wondering when the next emotional snipe was coming. The stress in the home continued, but not to the same extent.

The most surprising side effect of this chemo occurred about five days later when it felt like I went into menopause overnight. I experienced two days of constant hot flashes. It was physically and emotionally difficult because I was simultaneously having severe chills caused by the drug to increase my white blood cells. At one point, I was in bed under the electric blanket shivering for about two hours to increase my body temperature from 35° C to 36° C. I felt so sick. My torso was burning with hot flashes while the rest of me felt frozen. I continued to have hot flashes on a regular basis from the chemotherapy induced menopause, but never again like that weekend.

Monday was Thanksgiving Day, and it was wonderful. We visited a friend who had been diagnosed with colon cancer early that year, so she really understood what I was going through. She was so happy and grateful when we brought a present (a unique afghan I had been working on for about a year). After our visit, we came home and put the turkey in the oven. Eliza and I made the turkey dressing and Kevin agreed to stuff the turkey because I was afraid to handle raw meat. It was so funny when Kevin began to stuff the wrong end of the turkey; he had never heard of the Pope's nose before. We laughed and laughed. My nephew, niece and their one-year-old daughter Livvy came for dinner. I felt hopeful, and I prayed to see the next Thanksgiving.

As previously promised, I knew it was time to send a communication in order to keep everyone up to date on my progress. It was such a good idea to send a mass email to about forty people who I knew were thinking of me and wishing me well or praying for me. Using email helped me avoid being retraumatized from constantly repeating the information. This is the first one that I sent.

October 20, 2008

Hello Everyone:

I had promised to send out an email to tell everyone how I was doing, and I know that I have been a bit tardy. Life has been very busy and ever changing.

Just in case you do not know, I was diagnosed with advanced breast cancer in Aug. Life has a way of giving us very big surprises. Do not worry; just send your thoughts, prayers and any funny emails.

The cancer is very treatable even though the process will take at least ten months. Believe it or not, I have completed two chemo treatments. The chemo is working and the tumour is shrinking. I need to have six more chemo treatments. The next one is scheduled for Oct. 28. Hopefully, if everything stays on schedule I will be done early in Feb. I will be having a double mastectomy in March and radiation in April-May. Then in about one year, I plan to have two perky saline implants (gravity will never be a threat to me again).

It has been very hard on my family though. We have all had to change our ways of living.

I was started on what I consider a miracle drug (to stimulate my white blood cells because I was in trouble). I will find out on Friday if it worked but it is giving me some comfort and freedom in terms of infection. Leonie had strep throat last week and Kevin, Eliza and Leonie have all had colds.

The health unit and UWO have been great. I am working from home on my research, and I will not be teaching this year. How is that for flexibility? I would go crazy if I couldn't work.

I have experienced abundance in love and caring. I want to thank everyone for their thoughts cards and desserts for my girls and all other types of help.

It is nice when I hear from people. We are beginning a new life of cancer normal. I am very hopeful. I know that the chemo is saving my life and I welcome it.

I hope that you don't mind receiving news through a mass email because it is very hard to contact everyone individually.

Thanks again for thinking of me.

Hope that you are enjoying the fall.

Pat

The nice part about this method of communication was that so many people emailed me back and gave me words of encouragement. I was able to reread the messages and feel loved without getting overtired by talking on the phone. I also felt reaffirmed when so many people would mention the quality of my work.

Not all of my relationships survived this trauma in my life. I felt extremely hurt when a couple of long-term friends and family members could not be there for me. In both cases I felt deserted and betrayed. I was angry and heartbroken. I could not believe it was happening. I thought our relationships were almost sacrosanct and that they would always be there for me. I carried the shock of this for a long time even though there were many people who really cared. Old-time friends had deserted me when I needed them most. One of these friends did come and visit in October, and I now realize our friendship had been in trouble for a long time. I told her how angry and disappointed I was that she had not been in contact with me; she was angry over past unresolved conflicts. We agreed that day to start again, and there were a couple of phone calls from her, but she disappeared again and I have not heard from her since. Her family said she was having problems. I knew I no longer had the energy to pursue the relationship; it was another major loss in my life.

Kevin continued to be overwhelmed and stressed, and the fighting between he and Eliza returned with a vengeance. I asked Kevin (and he agreed) to begin counselling at the cancer clinic to help him cope with the family stresses, in particular his conflicts with Eliza. He attended the sessions, but I didn't see much more progress.

As fall arrived, I discovered I needed physical warmth.

We had our fireplace in the sunroom installed in early October. It made the room so welcoming and comfortable. Every day I would sit during in the sunroom and feel like I was outside without feeling cold. The fireplace was particularly special in the middle of the night because I would watch the fire in the darkness; it was like bringing light into a dark wilderness.

Chemo #3

By now, I was getting good at chemo time. I no longer got lost in the cancer clinic and could easily find where I had to go for all of my appointments. I was comforted at this pre-chemo appointment because my white blood cells were 3.3, well above the level required to receive chemo. This was such great news! Chemo 3 was uneventful as the symptoms occurred like clockwork. I didn't have as much indigestion, and no one was sick in the family.

Halloween has always been one of my favourite holidays. This year, Halloween happened on the Friday (five days after chemo). Unfortunately, I was too sick to answer the door to the trick or treaters, and I was still afraid of infection. I didn't have to put on a costume because I looked like a Halloween spectre: very pale, with very dark circles under my eyes. It was my facial appearance that made me feel very self-conscious. I looked a lot like Uncle Fester from the Addams Family. Kevin and the girls fulfilled the tradition of going over to Mary Poppins' home after trick or treating; I sighed and stayed home.

It was around this time I really began to notice that I was suffering from chemo brain. My brain was slower, I had difficulty concentrating and my ability to deal with stress plummeted. Thankfully, work was accommodating.

Ashley, my research assistant, was a tremendous help. We successfully submitted a couple of manuscripts, and the first workshop for the research grant was successful. I worked via teleconferences, or Ashley would come to my home. As much as I felt like my ability as a researcher was sliding, I wasn't prepared to give up. My work was too important, and I could cope, so long as I had support.

I continued to be hyper vigilant, watching and hoping that the tumour would shrink. I was filled with hope each time I could physically feel and see it getting smaller. I also remained hyper vigilant about avoiding sources of infection, knowing I could ill afford to have any of my chemo late because of a serious infection. I rarely went out anywhere in public, with the exception of my medical appointments and church. By the end of October, however, I was feeling socially isolated and decided to begin to have friends over to visit. We started having people visit during the second and third weeks after chemo, before the next dose. Everyone agreed not to come over if they were sick. People stayed about thirty to forty-five minutes so I didn't get overtired.

I also found that I was not immune to the stressors of life around me during chemo. At the end of October, I became more and more worried about one of my sisters. Unfortunately, Jean had become disabled in 2000, due to complications from abdominal surgery. She was now living in Michigan, and there had been many times over the past eight years that I felt the need to drop everything because she was seriously ill. I was upset because I realized I would not be able to go to her if she was ill. I called her and begged her to come to London; I even went to view apartments to entice her to come home. Unfortunately, my wishes were not hers. She decided to stay in Michigan.

During this chemo, Kate recommended I read a book by a former moderator of the United Church of Canada, *Postcards from the Valley*.[7] The book is about Rev. David Guiliano's journey with bone cancer. In the book, he described some of his suffering through multiple surgeries and radiation. He also continued to work through his treatments. The book was an inspiration to me and gave me hope that I also could make it.

Chemo #4

My fourth chemo was on my birthday. Kevin and I brought a carrot cake for the chemo staff, even though I couldn't eat sweets because they made me nauseous. The staff was most appreciative. My birthday treat was meeting a man in the waiting room who had come to the cancer clinic for his five-year follow-up appointment. He told us that five years before he had *seventy-six* tumours in his body and the doctors had given him six months to live. He requested chemo, but six months later nothing had changed. He then asked the doctors if there was anything else that could be done so he could have five more years of life. The doctors gave him another drug, and now he only had one very small tumour in his body. He smiled and told us, "Maybe I should have asked for ten years." I tell everyone this story. You just never know what will happen.

To my surprise, chemo four was much more difficult because of the cumulative effect of the drugs, which resulted in an increase in side effects. Earlier in November, we had planned for my sister to take the girls for the weekend so I could experience the side effects without having to worry about the girls' needs. Making the arrangements for the sleepover became stressful; first the sleepover was on, then it was off, and then it was on again and to be honest I can't even remember the reasons now. Kevin and I were looking forward to a relaxing weekend, but unfortunately, the time was not rejuvenating because the gastric symptoms were terrible on days five to seven. I had significant trouble eating and drinking because of the pain. About five days after the chemo, I also started having a feeling of over-whelming melancholy. I was tearful, irritable and panicky and had no idea why. I was so depressed and miserable for four days. Then on the fifth day, the melancholy lifted in what seemed like a few minutes. I talked to Lesley about it afterwards because we had both worked in psychiatric nursing for awhile. I said that it felt like a chemical depression because of the way it lifted so suddenly. She thought so as well. At the next chemo pre-appointment, I talked to my medical team about what happened. They thought the symptoms were caused by overexcitement from the large dose of steroid I had taken for the first three days and then withdrawal from the drug. Lesley asked me why I hadn't reached out earlier. I knew it was because I never would have asked for help in the past; I would never chance rejection while I was vulnerable. Would I reach out next time? I didn't think so.

The cumulative effect of the chemo was also evident when it took a longer time to physically recover from the fourth chemo, about two weeks instead of ten days. I managed to get on the stationary bike and elliptical trainer every day afterward, but I felt weak.

In November, Kevin's workload escalated. He is the administrator for a non-governmental agency and was currently working on a grant proposal. Because I have my PhD in program and policy evaluation, I tried to help him between bouts of nausea. Kevin felt guilty asking for my help, knowing I was so sick because I was also busy at the time preparing for a workshop. Most of the time work really did help me stay occupied, so I wouldn't think about dying as much, but this time I knew my abilities to produce were seriously compromised by chemo brain and the stress in my life.

About two weeks after the fourth chemo, I started worrying about the next chemo because I was starting a new regimen of drugs. (Apparently the cancer could adapt to the chemo and its potency could be reduced if more than four doses were given.) The side effects of the drug sounded like a nightmare: my blood pressure could fall; I had to wear ice mitts and ice boots so my nails wouldn't fall off; and there could be excruciating muscle and bone pain. I was relieved that the first four doses of chemo had worked because my tumour was now ten by twelve cm (about the size of a navel orange instead of a cantaloupe). Lynn told me the next chemo drugs could really shrink the tumour, but I continued to be frightened because I knew I still had a long way to go before the tumour was completely gone and the chemo side effects seemed very threatening.

I continued to pray that I would make it through the treatments. I began internalizing the imagery of some hymns. The hymn "On Eagle's Wings"[8] was particularly inspiring as I imagined God "raising me up on eagle's wings, carrying me on the breath of dawn, making me shine like the sun and holding me in the palm of his/her hands." We actually had a friend sing it as a solo at our wedding. Humming this hymn on the way to the pre-chemo appointment gave me the courage to tell the chemo nurse about my fears. She smiled gently and said. "We have been doing this a long time. Try and trust us to take care of you." I think God wanted me to meet her that day.

Chemo #5

Because of my trust in the chemo nurses, I found the courage to ask the nurse who would be giving this dose of chemo whether it would affect my heart. She said no; that was the previous chemo. I was so relieved I did not have that information when I was having the "red devil." The ice mitts and boots I wore to prevent my nails from falling off were very uncomfortable, but the sedative helped me to tolerate it; my blood pressure dropped a little but not seriously, and I was not nauseous. In contrast to the first regimen of chemo, I was now on double the amount of steroid to reduce the side effects and I began taking the steroids the day before chemo. Given my past history with the steroids, I was worried about getting more indigestion, but this side effect did not happen. I really had no side effects until the third night when I started to feel this "popping" feeling in my muscles. I didn't want to take any narcotics for muscle and bone pain because my thinking was already "screwed up" from the steroids, so I only took an over-the-counter pain medication. It helped a little. By the fourth day, the muscles in my tongue and neck didn't feel like they were working normally; my tongue felt "floppy," and there was a terrible metallic taste in my mouth that was not eradicated by food. I was warned again about the probability of mouth sores, but they didn't happen. By the sixth day, I felt terrible bone pain, and unfortunately Leonie was sick again. I was alone with the girls because Kevin had gone out for children's pain medication, and it seemed like he was gone for hours. The pain made moving difficult, and I could hardly stand while making supper. I tried walking the pain off, and it only became worse. My stomach bloated again, and food wouldn't digest; the inside of my mouth was like sandpaper, like, I imagine, the mouth of a cat. The symptoms ended on about the eighth day. I don't think this experience was ever as bad as the first chemo, but it was close.

Sometimes I made the mistake of viewing physical health problems as something to be tolerated because they were the result of the chemotherapy. One of these examples was the loss of some of my hearing. I hadn't been able to hear in my right ear for about two months. Therefore I decided to ask about the problem at my pre-chemo check up. Dr. B. (the general practitioner at the cancer clinic) examined my ear and, to my surprise, he said the problem was ear wax. I really felt silly thinking that something was the result of chemo and it was only ear wax. After the side effects of the chemo were primarily over, I decided to go to urgent care and get the problem addressed. Kevin dropped me off at the door of urgent care because Leonie was still feeling unwell. I sat alone in the hallway wearing a mask and feeling very conspicuous because the waiting room was full of very sick and contagious people. I kept repeating in my mind, "Please call my name so I can go home." Eventually, my name was called; the doctor syringed my ear and I went home to bed.

In early December, Kate had a Taize healing service during advent that Kevin and I attended. Taize is a service with many silences punctuated with chanting.

"Our darkness is never darkness in your sight:
The deepest night is clear as the daylight"[9]

It was a different spiritual service that was very moving. Kate handed out advent messages to the people who attended. My message read "Fast from doubt, feast on faith." Kevin's message said, "Fast from self-pity, feast on joy." We kept these sayings because they continued to be true and they were inspiring.

We were not immune to household mishaps during the treatment period, but the mishaps felt bigger in magnitude. For instance, we needed to get our furnace checked that week. The technician came and told me that our family might be in danger of carbon monoxide poisoning. I panicked because I was coming off the steroids. I asked the technician if he could change the furnace in the next few days. He said no, so I called his supervisor and explained I was very ill from chemo as a result of breast cancer and didn't need the additional stress of being terrified of carbon monoxide poisoning. The supervisor said the decision was up to the other worker. I was so angry that he was not more sensitive to my situation, especially given it was winter and we needed a functioning furnace to keep me warm. I called Hyde Park Heating and Cooling in London for help and started to cry on the telephone. I told him about my breast cancer and this supervisor kindly told me his sister and mother-in-law both had breast cancer and did "fine"; he said he would help me right away. I tell everyone about him! His kindness made all of the difference in the world to a person like me who felt like she was drowning.

That afternoon, I called my brother for some advice about the furnace because he is a licensed heating and ventilation worker. I felt a bit awkward on the phone because I had been feeling pretty cranky with him for not being more supportive of me during my treatment. There is nothing like desperation to initiate contact. To my delight, Bob came to London and looked at our furnace. He said the furnace would be able to make it until next summer. His visit gave me a feeling of both physical and emotional warmth and comfort.

The most significant change in my psyche after the symptoms of the fifth chemo were over was that I noticed I didn't feel like I was dying all of the time. It was such a relief to feel in my soul that my life was not slowly and surely leaving me. It was an early Christmas present for me.

Since we were children, my family has always celebrated Christmas Eve. I wanted to host Christmas at our house in the new sunroom, especially since I was unable to travel. We live in an area that has regular snowfalls while my brother and sister live in an area that receives less snow. My brother and sister worry about driving in snowy conditions more than Kevin and I do. This year I was really preoccupied with Christmas because I was still concerned that it would be my last. I found it stressful before Christmas because every time I talked to my siblings about coming for Christmas, they would respond "if the weather is good." Sometimes I felt angry because Kevin and I often travelled in rather poor weather conditions to be part of the family celebration. I began to resent my siblings for being worried about the weather when I was worried that this could be my last Christmas. It was very clear to me they were in denial about the seriousness of my illness and about what I felt was my probable death.

In the end, they all came and we celebrated Christmas Eve in our new sunroom. I helped prepare the Christmas dinner, but it was exhausting. At one point I just left and went to another area of the house to rest. We took a picture of my brother, my nephew and me because we were all bald. There is nothing like baldness to emphasize a family resemblance. That evening we went to the Christmas Eve service at Kate's church. It was so comforting and reassuring.

In the morning we opened a couple of presents. I had already given Kevin "two snow tires" (sung according to the "Twelve Days of Christmas") and Kevin gave me "two snow tires." The girls opened their gifts. Due to my chemo brain, I couldn't actually remember where I had put one of Eliza's presents. It became a bit of joke because Leonie, the most gifted child in the world for finding things, travelled through the house and found it. I felt very grateful to her.

Chemo #6

My next chemo was planned between Christmas and New Year's Eve. Since this is a period of lower levels of staffing at the chemo clinic, I was fine with the decision to go straight to chemo without seeing my oncology team. Nevertheless, just before Christmas, I became upset when the cancer clinic called to ask whether my appointment could be moved from the Monday prior to New Year's Eve to New Year's Eve. I felt upset by this request because I wanted to go to the wedding of a very good friend (Poole) on February 14th and I didn't want any of my chemo treatments delayed. In the end, I agreed to change the date because I knew the request meant that someone from out of town needed to have chemo treatment at that time, maybe someone just like me.

Rearranging the scheduled chemo turned out for the best. There was such a holiday spirit at the clinic on New Year's Eve. While overall I did not find the chemo clinic a dismal place, on this day people seemed to be laughing and joking more than usual. The chemo itself was uneventful, and amazingly, I wasn't even as worried about reacting to the drug.

New Year's Eve was pretty quiet at our house as I was glad to see 2008 leave, hoping for a better 2009. It was comforting to know I only had two more chemo treatments to go! Since women with non-advanced chemo usually only have six doses, I knew I would have been finished my chemo if I didn't have locally advanced breast cancer. My situation was different though. I still could feel the tumour (eleven cm by ten cm), but it was smaller and now felt spongy rather than like one big lump. My oncologist's nurse practitioner, Lynn, told me that the tumour was supposed to disintegrate from the inside out now. I could feel this happening.

After my sixth chemo, I sent out another mass email to update people on my progress.

January 7 09
Hello Everyone:

I can't believe 2009 has finally come to greet us all. For me, it feels like a new year of healing.

I have finished six doses of chemo now, only two to go. The chemo has definitely worked. I am not really sure how big the tumour is at this point. That is such a big change from a cantaloupe.

The fourth chemo was rather hard because there was a cumulative effect. The fifth was also a bit hard because it was a new drug, but six was much better. I think that I am actually healing from the first four because I now have a layer of lamb's wool hair on my head. No more drafts. I can now bend over and not have my hat fall in my eyes. I am back to only one hat on my head, rather than two.

I have a surgeon's appointment on Feb. 4th. I hope that my last chemo occurs on Feb. 5 and then surgery the first week of March. I have a bit of cabin fever, but I have white blood cells for 5 days every three weeks, so I am pretty grateful for them.

Most people think that I am very optimistic and courageous. I want you all to know that I am still the same old endearing wimp as in the past. Perhaps I will be offered a Hollywood contract after all of this is over. Someone asked me, "Wasn't I glad that 2008 was over?" (like it was a bad year). I would like to clarify for everyone that restarting my dissertation with only eight months to go was by far a more stressful year. Everything is quite relative, isn't it.

We had a really nice Christmas. I want to thank everyone for all of the visits and cards and prayers. I have been tripping over the abundance in my life. Leonie has finally settled down, which is quite a relief. Kevin is still pretty busy with work.

Please keep me in your prayers. I still have another five months to go before the radiation is all over.

My family thinks this is a nice letter.

May 2009 keep you well and happy.

Pat

Kevin and I continued to be concerned about Leonie. She was constantly unwell and stressed. She was having problems with school work and had missed about half of her school time by now. Luckily her teacher was very understanding. Her stress was also affecting her friendships, and conflicts were occurring. She worried that I was dying, and her friends were deserting her.

Kevin and I decided that Leonie needed more support from her friends, so we decided to organize some sleepovers when she agreed to some ground rules. The girls had to be in bed by 11:00 p.m., and they couldn't disturb me. In addition, they could not come over if they were sick. Leonie now had friends over most weekends except during my chemo treatments. As a result, life was at times more cheerful for Leonie.

Chemo #7

Chemo number seven was completely uneventful. The only thing I noticed was that my muscles stayed sore longer than they had during the previous chemos. I was very proud of the few strands of hair that had started to grow on my head in January, even before all the chemo treatments were over. I wondered, *Does this mean my body is healing in spite of the physical assault of chemo and the emotional and family chaos?*

Meanwhile, I continued work on my research even though my chemo brain was just as pronounced as ever. Gayle in human resources at the health unit wanted me to complete long-term disability papers just in case I could not return to work full time. I reluctantly started the paperwork. Gayle was so kind and supportive to me, but I just didn't want to mentally think of myself as disabled.

Chemo #8

The day before my last chemo, I met with Dr. Holiday (my surgeon) about my upcoming surgery. I would be booked for the pre-operative appointment later in the month. I felt confident that Dr. Holiday and Pat (his nurse practitioner) would take good care of me.

February 5, 2008: the last day of my chemo finally arrived. I am sure that many cancer patients are jubilant when this day finally arrives. I found waiting for this day agonizing, and I was a bit fearful as well. I knew that after this chemo was over, there would only be the surgery and radiation treatments to stop the cancer from returning. Chemo attacked any cancer throughout the body, whereas surgery and radiation are local treatments. I now had to believe that if there were any leftover rogue cancer cells in my body beyond my breast, my immune system would have to stop them. I was worried, however, because I was not sure my body had the physical resilience to fight after being so compromised from all of the chemo.

In order to prepare me for my last chemo, I asked Kate to come and serve me communion at home. I wanted to find the strength to have the final chemo four days early so I could go to Poole's wedding February 14th. I knew the chemo might be much harder on my body because I was having it earlier than usual. I thought the most potent protection I could have was communion served just to me, and it was such a healing experience. I have never felt so important as an individual, and I gained strength knowing that this communion was being prepared just for me. Kate also used the laying on of spiritual hands. I felt very strong and much of my tearfulness, doubts and fears abated.

When I arrived at the chemo clinic for my last dose, I told the person who took my blood that it was my last round of chemotherapy treatment. I told strangers in the clinic hall it was my last chemo. I had witnessed so many people make the same comments ahead of me when I was in the early stages of chemo; now it was my turn.

I didn't worry too much about my blood work because I felt pretty confident it would be fine and the chemo would proceed and it did. I can remember what happened as if it was yesterday. The beeper vibrated. It was time. A familiar nurse who had given me about four of my treatments came up, greeted me and brought me to the back chemo room without windows, which I didn't mind. When she found out it was my last chemo, she rearranged her assignment and actually ended up starting the IV and giving me the chemo. It made the experience feel supportive and familiar. When my chemo was over, I rang the bell at reception that a child had donated to the chemo clinic to help people mark the important milestone of having their last treatments. The music was positively delightful!

When I returned home from my final treatment, I decided to make some changes to the plan for coming off of the steroid. Since I had accidentally forgotten to take a dose last time, I couldn't see any reason why I shouldn't taper myself more slowly off the steroid. As a result, I only had a few of the emotional symptoms of steroid withdrawal.

I wondered if the side effects from chemo would be different since I went for the treatment early, and they were. On the fourth day, I felt a tingling in my hands and feet that affected my balance and strength. I had heard about this symptom from others and knew it could happen. I decided that since it was my last chemo, I would stay in bed and take the anti-inflammatory medication every eight hours instead of every twelve hours. I didn't want this symptom to get out of hand. Little did I know that I would have neuropathy (damage to nerves causing pain, numbness and tingling in my feet and hands) for the next nine months.

Luckily, I had finished much of the academic work on the research grant prior to the chemo, so I wasn't feeling pressured at work. My research assistant was right "on the ball," because I received a phone call to gently remind me that I had completely forgotten to send in an acceptance to a conference. I asked Laura to complete this acceptance for us because it was difficult to type with the tingling in my fingers, and she did.

Leonie fared much better after I finished this chemo. Leonie did not realize the change in date for the treatment because my chemo was early, so consequently she did not get upset in advance. She was so relieved when I told her my last chemo treatment was over. I am positive this was the first true relief she had since my chemo began. She did not experience any stomach aches, nervousness and difficulty sleeping during this last round of chemo.

As Poole's wedding approached, I started thinking more about my appearance. Even though my hair was starting to grow back, I did not have any eyebrows or eyelashes by this point. The week before Poole's wedding, I went to my hairstylist, Farzaneh, to get my eyebrows dyed onto my face so I would look more "normal." I knew my ability to pencil them on would be limited. People warn you about trying to dye your hair when having chemo treatments, and they are right. Farzaneh tried to dye my eyebrows on once, but the dye didn't work. She darkened the dye solution and tried again. Eliza and Leonie were laughing because I looked sinister. Again and again the dye didn't work. This visit became a source of entertainment rather than beauty.

Despite the challenges, I went to Poole's wedding just as I wanted. I hobbled into the building, and I had to wear two hats because of the cold of winter. My eyes had been weeping constantly for the past three days before the wedding and now they were really itchy. It was like old times when we got to the wedding early and I saw Poole's parents.

"Hello Sealy," Poole greeted me and looked at my eyebrows and said she thought I had told her I did have any eyebrows. I started to laugh and told Poole that I drew them on. She laughed and told me she was wearing old contacts. I said everyone would be thinking I was crying because she was getting married when it was really my lack of eyelashes that caused me to weep. You can say these things when you have been friends for almost thirty years. Poole told me that her husband-to-be Kip was touched that I would have chemo early so I could still come to their wedding. I felt my heartstrings pull. Even though Kevin and I left before dinner, I was really glad I was able to help my friend celebrate her wedding.

The following week, we went out as a family to attend a Shrove Tuesday pancake supper at Kate's church. My efforts to go out were really rewarded because I saw two of my friends there. We only stayed about one hour, but that was enough for me. The evening was great. I felt like I was reconnecting with my friends, and perhaps the worst was over.

After the chemo treatments were over, the main issue was dealing with the knowledge that I now had to fight the cancer myself. I knew I still needed to reduce my stress. Work was under control, but my family was still very emotionally draining. I continued to struggle with issues from my past, especially around having to be independent and responsible at a very young age. I knew I was being overprotective of my children, and sometimes I would rationalize that my illness was forcing the girls to be more responsible for themselves. It was challenging, however, for my family to increase their domestic responsibilities and emotionally comfort themselves. On one hand, I was aware of the anger and resentment I felt, because it seemed I was constantly taking care of Kevin and the girls while neglecting myself; however, on the other hand, I still had trouble letting go. I wondered if I could ever heal if I didn't get enough peace and rest. For the first time, I told my family I had "done" things for everyone much longer than maybe I should have. I really started talking about how everyone needed to be more responsible doing his or her chores, so I could heal. I wanted them to hear me, but they were too stressed to hear. Nothing changed. My reality was that no one changed overnight.

Having cancer treatment means you know quite well that others are also having cancer treatment. Three people I knew from the psychiatric hospital where I had previously worked (Susan, Eric and Larry) also had cancer at the same time as me. I would often ask Lesley how they were doing, but when you have cancer, people naturally want to protect you from upsetting news. Susan fought lung cancer for almost a year, but unfortunately she died of a brain tumour in February. The first I knew of her death was when I read it in the obituaries. Eric also died of leukemia. I grieved for the family, and I was afraid for myself. Larry had a very serious leukemia and believe it or not, he is surviving against the odds. I sincerely do not understand why some people get cancer and others don't. I also don't understand who survives and who doesn't. It is a terrible mystery for me. It is probably a terrible mystery for everyone.

At the end of February, we had a "Madame Curie" (discoverer of radiation) ham and bean soup party for our friends who were going to drive me to the radiation clinic. It was a great evening even though I sat in a chair most of the night because it was too painful to walk. We could see a crescent moon with a halo out of the sunroom window. It was both mysterious and comforting.

Reflections:

- Our world revolved around the chemo time. Approximately one week of symptoms, one week of recovery, and one week to get ready for the next dose.
- I treated chemo just as I did communion. I prayed and invited it to make me whole. It was emotionally traumatic to have to wait and pray each day hoping that the tumour would shrink just a little more.
- The drug that increases white blood cells made all the difference in the world because none of my chemo treatments were delayed because my white cells were too low. It was somewhat reassuring to know I would have white blood cells five days every three weeks. It allowed me maintain better contact with people I care about.
- I felt safe having people come to my house. No one visited while they were ill.
- I was very fortunate to have as few side effects from chemo as I did. I wasn't in real trouble from the side effects until the last chemo.
- It felt very comforting to begin losing the feeling I was dying, but I still carried the fear.
- Journaling was helpful because it allowed me to pour out my thoughts, especially my fears.

- Leonie was especially traumatized by the chemotherapy. I am not sure anything really comforted her.
- I really wish that Kevin, Eliza and Leonie could have been more self-sufficient.
- I was angry and resentful that suffering with chemo was enough without the burden of all of the family's problems. I should have reached out for more help from my friends.
- Holidays gain more importance because you wonder if it is the last time you will experience them.
- Some family and friends will not be able to rise to the occasion. It can lead to feelings of betrayal.
- Work helped me keep a functional part of my identity so I didn't feel completely disabled, and it diverted me from my fears of death. I was very fortunate to be a researcher with an understanding employer.
- It was still very hard to tell my close friends everything because I did not want to be a burden. I knew they were also worried that I may not make it.
- Weekly church services with communion helped to ground and heal me.
- Praying for others was easy, and I felt that God would listen and help. Praying for myself was very difficult, and I doubted whether I would be heard. It was clear I didn't trust God to help me as much as I trusted God to help others.

Chapter 3

Good Friday: Double Mastectomy

My double mastectomy occurred during Lent; in fact, I thought it was a good omen to have surgery on the World Day of Prayer, March 6, 2009. I had experienced much suffering in life, but the complications from my surgery led me to a whole new level of vulnerability.

A sword pierced Jesus' side even though he was probably already dead. A scalpel severed off my breasts, but I was anesthetized.

After surgery I felt a bit like Peter. He was so self-assured that he would never deny Jesus. I never dreamt that I would have complications. Peter denied Jesus three times and then he wept. I had three major complications: hemorrhage, sepsis and radiation burn, and I also wept.

Given my anxious personality, it was fortunate I was in denial that my double mastectomy was major surgery. To my surprise, I didn't start worrying about the surgery until the middle of February, about three weeks before the surgical date. First I worried that my white blood cells and platelets (blood cells that cause clotting) would be depressed, which would preclude surgery. I still could feel the tumour, so delaying surgery would mean I would be at risk of the tumour growing again.

Kevin and I went to the pre-operative appointment at the end of February. It was a very cold day, so Kevin dropped me off at the door of the hospital. I still had marked difficulty walking because of the neuropathy (pain and numbness) in my hands and feet. Luckily my eyes were no longer watering every minute from my lack of eyelashes. I felt very self-conscious because I looked very sick and I was convinced people in the lobby and hallway were staring at me.

The first part of the pre-operative appointment was obtaining my physical information. My weight was up because of the steroids, and I felt bloated, bald and ugly! I was also worried the electrocardiogram (EKG) would detect heart problems from the side effects of the chemo, which could mean my surgery could be postponed, but it was fine. I also met individually with a pre-op nurse who went over the surgical day procedures and post-operative care. First, there were the pre-op instructions: nothing to eat or drink after midnight, but it was okay to take my sedative with a mouthful of water. I didn't want to embarrass myself by crying hysterically if I got scared as I had prior to other surgeries. I was warned to watch for post-operative complications, such as bleeding and infection. I really wasn't worried about these side effects because I was too busy being worried I would die from the anesthetic, which was highly unlikely since I had had previous anesthetics without complications. The nurse gave me two pink pillows to rest my arms on after surgery because I would have two portable suction drains (one on each side). In parting, the nurse said "Don't forget your pillows on the surgical day."

It is still shocking that my double mastectomy was out-patient day surgery. I asked about whether I could stay the night, but this meant the surgery would be postponed until there was an available bed. I was too afraid to take that risk because I didn't want the tumour growing again. An advantage of day surgery was that the risk of catching a hospital-acquired infection was lower. I would take my chances with outpatient surgery!

Chronology of Medical Appointments and Family Activities:
March 6 to March 26, 2009

Sunday	Monday	Tuesday	Wednesday	Thursday	Friday	Saturday
					March 6 - 8:30 am: Surgery 12:45 pm: Surgery over 4:00 pm: Home 9:00 pm: Bleed	March 7 - 2:00 pm: Emergency Room visit
March 8 - 3:00 am: surgical drain detaches 1:00 pm: Jodi leaves 6:45 pm: Karen arrives			March 11 - Dr. Holiday	March 12 - My drain site begins to hurt		

March 6 to March 26, 2009 - continued

Sunday	Monday	Tuesday	Wednesday	Thursday	Friday	Saturday
March 15 - 8:00 am: Chills begin but no fever 2:00 pm: Fever of 37.6° 3:30 pm: Emergency Room Visit; Admitted in the middle of the night	March 16 - 9:00 am: Dr. Holiday removes the drains Home on oral antibiotics 7:00 pm: Chills, back to Emergency 10:00 pm: Kevin leaves	March 17 - 6:00am: Admitted to the hospital Find out I am septic and will stay for a few days in the hospital. Eliza and Leonie are very worried			March 20 - 1:00 pm: IV interstitial (not working) 3:00 pm: New IV and I go home	
March 22 - IV interstitial and replaced in a previous vein. Very painful		March 24 - IV out	March 25 - Dr. Holiday pathology report			

In February, my friend Jodi, who has been my friend since our first year of university (almost thirty years), offered to take care of me at home after the day surgery, even when it meant taking time off of work and travelling from Peterborough to London. I agreed with a grateful heart because I knew I would be safe with Jodi taking care of me. Michelle, my niece, also offered to take a day off of work and take care of Eliza and Leonie during my surgery and then overnight. I was so grateful I burst into tears because I didn't want the girls at home to see me the night after surgery.

I took a sedative the night before surgery and slept. Originally I had to be at the hospital at 6:30 a.m. for the 8:00 a.m. operation, but the schedule was changed. Dr. Holiday decided to operate on someone else before me. At the time of my surgery, Dr. Holiday was primarily doing mastectomies. There was something comforting about knowing another person was "in my boat," perhaps not as sick as I was.

On the day of the surgery, Michelle arrived at our house at 7:45 a.m. to get the girls. I put on a brave face as Kevin and I said goodbye to Eliza and Leonie and left for the hospital. We arrived at 8:30 a.m., and a friendly nurse greeted me. She looked great. She was a godsend because she told me she had survived breast cancer after having a double mastectomy. She told me she had completed breast reconstruction about three years before. WOW! It is worth repeating that she really looked great. You would never know she had been through so much just by looking at her. Meeting her before my surgery gave me such a surge of hope!

I barely got changed into my hospital gown when Dr. Holiday came into my bed bay. His previous surgery had finished earlier than planned. He said, "Come now." I was so busy being impressed with the health of my nurse that I didn't even have a chance to get scared. A porter came and took me to the operating room where I waited in the hallway outside of the surgical suite (clearly not as nice as a hotel suite). The anesthetist greeted me, brought me into the operating room and put in the IV for the anesthetic. I was not anxious since the surgical staff was still busy preparing the operating room for the surgery. I felt relaxed thinking there was still time before anything serious happened. Then the anesthetist told me my arm was going to feel warm and it did; that was the last thing I remembered until I awoke in the recovery room. I actually went to sleep without fear; what a blessing! Imagine the surgery being just over two hours and waking up with no memory of it happening. The first thing I remember was the recovery nurse trying to wake me up, asking, "Are you in pain?" I said no, but she gave me some pain medication to help me be more comfortable on the stretcher ride back to the outpatient area.

The original nurse who had breast reconstruction surgery greeted me when I returned to the outpatient area. She came into my room and helped me onto my day bed and made me comfortable. Now I am not exactly sure if I dreamed this or not, but I remember my nurse asking me if I wanted to see her reconstructed breast. I said yes. She pulled the curtain around the bed and let me feel her breast. It felt like a twenty-five-year-old breast. She told me it was an implant that goes under the muscle so it feels firm. There was no way for me to really tell if this memory was real or imagined. The memory is still vivid and still fills me with hope.

About 3:30 p.m., it was time to get ready to go home. Before I left the hospital, I had to go to the bathroom. I struggled and strained to get up. I never realized how difficult it would be to move with two surgical drains attached to my chest. After Kevin finished talking to the Community Care Access Center coordinator who was arranging home nursing care, Kevin and I left for home. A community nurse would be scheduled to visit the next day.

By the time we arrived home, Jodi was waiting for us. Kevin walked behind me as I climbed the stairs to our bedroom. I didn't want him to touch me for fear I would get hurt if my arms were accidentally pulled. I wanted to be independent: "I can do the stairs by using my own two legs." I didn't feel any pain. Little did I know that the nerves were cut and I wouldn't be feeling anything for many months to come.

That night I noticed a hematoma (a bleed under the skin) forming on the left side of my chest. My mind was foggy; what was I supposed to do? The hematoma lump began as the size of a pea on my non-cancerous left side and grew to the size of a golf ball. I called the surgical resident twice but no one answered my call. I was afraid to move and possibly make it worse. I lay awake all night because I didn't want to bleed to death while sleeping. I felt abandoned by the medical system when no doctors or nurses returned my phone calls. It never occurred to me to call Dr. Holiday, probably because the pain medication was interfering with my thinking. If he knew, he would have helped me.

The next morning I was still worried. The lump was smaller, but a bruise was forming that was about 25 cm by 25 cm (see the picture). We called the visiting nurse, but she didn't return my call in the morning even though I left about four messages on the answering service. Kevin left around noon to pick up Eliza and Leonie and take them to the hotel room where they were staying overnight. The visiting nurse came in the afternoon. I asked, "Should I go to the emergency room?" She agreed it was a big bruise and said to go "If it would make you feel more comfortable." I was still frightened, and so we went.

It was pouring rain when Jodi drove me to the emergency department. Jodi dropped me off at the door because I could hardly walk. People were staring, and I knew I looked really bad. The nurses did not make me wait in the waiting room. I was directed to the psychiatric bed bay where there were no patients at that moment. One doctor examined me, then decided to get a consult from the surgical fellow (next level up in the hierarchy of doctors). The surgical resident said, "No, you are okay, the bruise will go down." The surgical drains on each side were working fine. Jodi and I drove home. By now it had rained so much that water washed over the top of the car as we drove over deep puddles.

The water going over the car did not feel like a normal baptism. It was more like a baptism by fire.

When we got home, Jodi made us dinner and I went to bed. The night was uneventful until about 3:00 a.m. when I woke up laying in a pool of blood. The surgical drain on the right side (the cancerous side) had detached. I started to cry and called out to Jodi, and she came to me right away. We tried to clean the end of the drain tubes the best we could and put them back together. Jodi was successful, and I fell back to sleep.

The visiting nurse came daily for the next few days. She changed my dressing because there was old blood everywhere on the right chest dressing. While she was changing the dressing, I realized that the days of sterile technique were over. In the past, nurses would use sterile gloves and sterile solution while cleaning a wound. Now, the nurse used clean technique instead that involves using clean, but not sterile, gloves and a special cleaning solution. I wondered out loud about getting an infection, but the nurse said "Everything will be fine."

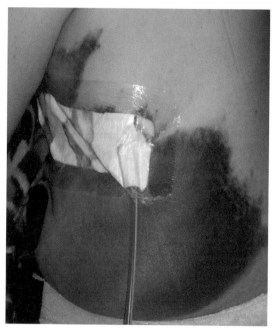

I bled the night of the surgery at home. This is a picture of the bruise from the hematoma about one week after surgery. You can see some of the bruise beginning to lighten at the top. The old blood sank down towards my waist. I had the bruise for about one month. The plastic tube is the drain that was inserted at surgery. There were about 120 cc (4 oz.) of old blood coming out from the drain every day after the hematoma.

By the second postoperative day, I was only capable of walking very slowly to the bathroom and the sunroom. Jodi and I talked about old times. It was so reassuring to have her with me, and I started to cry when she had to leave on Sunday. Jodi did make things "safe" and loving for me. I was glad to see Kevin and Eliza and Leonie when they came home Sunday afternoon. Given what happened, it was a very good decision not to let the girls see me in the first couple of days after my surgery. I was also very fortunate my friend Karen arrived from Toronto that afternoon to stay with me until Wednesday. I knew before surgery I wouldn't want to be alone during the day when Kevin was at work. I knew we all needed Karen's support.

Unlike Jesus' disciples, Jodi and Karen were there to comfort and take care of me. They were there when I called.

The next few postoperative days were uneventful, once I adjusted to the sleep deprivation from having to lay on my back because of the surgical drains. I had an uncomfortable abrasive feeling lower down across my ribs where Dr. Holiday must have scraped off the breast tissue, but I rarely took the pain medication because I was numb from along the incision line and through to the right armpit.

On Wednesday (my fifth post-operative day), I met with Dr. Holiday for a follow-up appointment; however, on Thursday, my right drain started hurting. I asked the visiting nurse, "Can the drain come out yet?" She replied, "No, not until the drainage is less than thirty cc over twenty-four hours." The drain hurt more the next day and even more the day after that. In hindsight, I should have called Dr. Holiday. We didn't, and that was a very a big mistake.

On Sunday morning (nine days postoperative), I woke up feeling a terrible chill. I just couldn't get warm. My temperature was 37° C, but my normal temperature was usually about 36.5°C. A couple of hours later, I was really shaking and my temperature increased to 37.6°C. Luckily, I remembered Dr. Potvin's advice about infection. I thought if my platelets didn't work sufficiently to prevent hemorrhage (even though the quantity was sufficient), then maybe my white blood cells probably wouldn't work either. I was worried, so I asked Kevin to take me to the emergency room at 3:30 p.m.

Kevin called Lesley to come over and help with the girls while we were at the emergency room. When we arrived, everyone stared because I looked even more ill than when I hemorrhaged. A staff member looked at me incredulously and said, "You mean you had a double mastectomy as outpatient?" My heart rate was very high (148 beats per minute as compared to the normal 60 to 100 beats per minute) and my blood pressure was low. The doctors thought I had an infection. (Damn the tube that fell apart.) The nurse took blood cultures, and I went for a chest x-ray. I was so cold, deathly cold. I felt panicky when I remembered, from my days as an intensive care nurse, that people with septic shock often die. The medical team started IV antibiotics and infused litres of IV fluid. Thank God I was admitted to the hospital because we never would have been able to cope with my illness at home. After a couple of hours, I felt much better. The next morning, Dr. Holiday came in to see me and he took out my surgical drains. I was going to be started on oral antibiotics and I could go home. I really wanted to go home. The nurse looked incredulous when she heard the news and said "Shouldn't she stay another day?" Dr. Holiday said that I could go home because I was doing so much better. This nurse may have been a prophet.

Later that day at 4:00 p.m., the chills came again. We called Lesley again to come over and help, but she could only stay at our house until 10:00 p.m. This time my experience at the emergency room was frightening. The resident on duty minimized my problems, and I was neglected. Most of the nurses and doctors seemed to be chatting about their social life or work complaints, instead of taking care of the patients. When Kevin helped me to the bathroom, a gush of old blood came out from the left side where I had the original bleed, and I started to cry. No one responded to ask me what was wrong. No one asked if I had taken my regular dose of oral antibiotics; no one gave me any IV antibiotics. I just lay there on the stretcher feeling frantic. It was clear to me I had a serious infection. At 10:00 p.m., Kevin had to leave and go home to the girls. I felt so alone. I didn't feel like the emergency room team even noticed my distress or cared that I was upset. I stayed agitated throughout the night, feeling all alone, wondering if I would die of sepsis (bacteria in the blood).

At 6:00 a.m. the next morning (eleventh post-operative day), I was once again admitted to the hospital to the gynecology wing and started on IV antibiotics. I still felt hysterical from my treatment through the night. When the nurse helped me into bed, I started to sob and shed the tears of desperation and hopelessness that I had stored up over the past six months. The nurse listened to me with the most empathetic eyes. I told her of my fear of dying like my mother and abandoning my girls. I talked about having to take care of my family and not having the time to take care of myself. I sobbed some more, literally crying for about half an hour before I fell asleep. The kind nurse awoke me around noon because I had to move to another room. She helped me shower first, and I showed her my bruise only to discover the old blood had leaked all over my clothes again. She helped me dress. I felt love for that nurse, and it felt like she saved me. Then I had to leave for another room.

My new room was right beside the nurses' station. I was amazed that a patient could hear so much information about others as the nurses talked in the nurses' station. It was more distressing to hear them talk about me. It turned out that my haemoglobin level was low, probably from the bleed and the significant amount of IV fluid that I had received. I figured that I would be okay because I usually ate foods rich in iron in my diet. That afternoon I found out I had been septic (gram positive bacillus), and I would be staying in the hospital on IV antibiotics for a few more days.

Being in the hospital was even more difficult because Eliza and Leonie were very upset I had to stay in the hospital during March break. They had tears in their eyes when they came to visit every day, and I knew they were wondering if I was going to die. I told them that the medicine was working, but I would not be home for a few days.

That night (twelfth postoperative day) when I got up to go to the bathroom, I felt another tear on my right side just above the incision line. I got another hematoma; this one was also the size of a golf ball, but I didn't worry about it like I had about the previous one. I felt that it wouldn't be the thing that would kill me.

My biggest fear while in the hospital shifted to the fragility of my veins since I was not allowed to have blood work in my right arm because of the lymph node resection (the removal of the lymph nodes by my armpit). A tourniquet could put unnecessary stress on the lymphatic system on my right arm, which could cause lymphedema (swelling of the arm because of inadequate lymph drainage). Just as I had feared, my current IV went interstitial (stopped working) and needed to be restarted. I felt afraid when my nurse in the hospital admitted to me she was not very experienced at starting IVs. My fear turned to frustration and anger when she tried unsuccessfully to begin the IV. I felt she should have called the IV team before trying herself, especially given her inexperience. The IV team nurse successfully put in the IV, but the only vein was very small. I thought, *Oh right, how long will this vein last before it breaks?* After four days in the hospital, I went home on IV antibiotics. As I was leaving, I saw an elderly church member who volunteered at the hospital. Even though she was close to being ninety years old, she looked so spry compared to me. I will never forget that feeling of vulnerability.

At home, I moved from fretting about dressings and emptying surgical drains to worrying about the IV medication. I watched each dose go in my last remaining vein hoping and praying the vein would not go interstitial. One of my biggest irritations during this period was that I never knew when the community nurses would show up. It was a different time every day, and I wondered, would my IV stop before they came? Yes, it did. The visiting nurse reinserted the IV very close to where it had been previously because there were no other working veins, but the IV site hurt. The vein lasted until the end of the IV therapy, but it really hurt by the time my last dose of antibiotics came due. I called the visiting nurses many times and didn't get an answer so I left a message. My patience was gone; I cried hysterically as I repeatedly tried to telephone the home care office without an answer. The last dose of antibiotics successfully went into the vein, but it hurt a lot. The nurse came a few hours later and took out the hated IV. I sometimes wish I could have taken it out myself, but I could only use one hand and I had no feeling in my fingers. Each extra day of suffering further exhausted me physically and emotionally. I had lost twenty pounds, looked and felt dreadful, but I survived this traumatizing experience.

The same day that I went septic, a dear friend was in a life and death situation suffering from a brain injury. When I found out, Kevin took some of our home-made frozen meals to his wife Anna. Although difficult, we knew my surgery was going to happen, whereas they were thrown into a frightening situation out of the blue. We didn't tell them about my sepsis until everyone was confident that our friend would survive. I felt sorry for Lesley because now two of her friends were in life and death situations.

No one is immune to life and death situations. We just think that things are fine because nothing has happened yet. I bet the disciples had no idea the Pharisees were coming when they went to sleep while Jesus was praying in Gethsemane.

Twenty days after my surgery, I had an appointment with Dr. Holiday to review the pathology report. My world seemed to stop or whirl as I heard the results. The good news was that the chemo had worked and shrunk the tumour to five cm; the bad news was that ten out of twelve lymph nodes were positive for cancer. I automatically jumped to the conclusion the cancer was going to come back. Did this mean I was dying? Dr. Holiday and Pat both said, "No one really knows." Some people have no positive lymph nodes and the cancer returns. Some people live for twenty or more years with positive lymph nodes and die from another ailment. My fear escalated after this appointment, so after a few days I called Dr. Potvin's clinic and told Lynn (Dr. Potvin's nurse practitioner) just how frightened I was. She explained the lymph nodes were viewed in a chain for the pathology report which to me meant that at least there were two lymph nodes that were cancer free between the cancer and the rest of my body. Even though I was afraid, I tried to hold onto that thought.

April Fool's Day was pleasantly memorable this year, because Dr. Holiday told me he would not need to aspirate the second hematoma; it could resolve on its own. This was the first really positive news I felt in a long time. Another stage of treatment was over.

Reflections:

- The pre-operative system worked great. It was nice of them to give me those specially designed pink pillows.
- Even though it was nice to come home and be in my own bed after surgery, I wish could have stayed as an inpatient the first night. Hemorrhaging was very stressful on top of everything else. Given the amount of chemo I had, perhaps it wasn't surprising my platelets didn't work. I didn't need the stress of having to go home when I really didn't have full function of both arms.
- Thank you, Michelle, for taking care of my kids. I didn't need the stress of trying to reassure them. I am very glad

A Family's Resurrection from Breast Cancer

that they didn't see me right after surgery. I could never have reassured them that night and day.

- The health care system needs to respond better to women in my condition, especially post-surgically. To make patients wait for surgery in order to be an inpatient doesn't feel like a choice.

- I was very glad that Jodi was there with me, especially when I bled. What do non-nurses do when they see the drain has detached and blood is flowing everywhere?

- I was very impressed with most of the ER and inpatient staff my first night. I was really unimpressed with the ER staff the second night. Their behaviour was really as different as day and night. The second night was one of the most frightening nights of my life while I had to listen to their idle chatter and laughter. Even though I had been a director of nursing for over seventeen years, I didn't file a complaint. I was just too tired and despondent.

- I am very grateful to the nurse in the hospital who listened to me sob for at least half an hour while she made me feel like I was her only patient and had all the time in the world to take care of me. I hope this isn't a rare occurrence among nurses.

- Home care needs to be improved. At a bare minimum, a nurse should have visited me the first night. They need to tell the patients when they are coming so there isn't as much uncertainty about their arrival.

- I wonder if using sterile technique (rather than clean technique) to change my dressing would have prevented the infection. I should have called Dr. Holiday when my drain was becoming progressively more painful. I just didn't think of it.

100

- Sepsis was by far the worst experience of my cancer treatment. *For me, it was 3:00 p.m. on the afternoon of Good Friday.*
- Sometimes you are so sick that you cannot even think of relationships and emotional well-being.
- Imagine what would have happened without the prayers of everyone who cared about me.

Chapter 4

Good Friday: Radiation

We don't know if it was sunny on the day that Jesus was crucified. If it was, he would have been burnt in the sun. He said, "I am thirsty." He was given vinegar. My skin was burnt with radiation. It became parched and bled and wept; I bathed it with Epsom salts.

Easter Sunday weekend occurred during my first week of radiation. This Easter I sincerely prayed to Jesus, who healed the sick, to save me. I had never used the word "save" until then. I thought of it often after that experience.

It is hard to believe I started radiation one month after the surgery and about two weeks after being discharged from the hospital after being septic (infection in my skin area that resulted in infection in the blood). I was exhausted and wanted to postpone the radiation until I had healed more, but I was afraid that the cancer would come back. I knew from Dr. Pereira (the radiation oncologist) that I would be having thirty doses of radiation over a five-week period (Monday to Friday).

In early April, Kevin took me to the radiation clinic for my pre-radiation tattoos. I had never been tattooed before. I always thought tattoos were supposed to be fun, but mine weren't. My tattoos were a series of little dots on my chest that were pretty far apart. One of the tattoos hurt a lot as the needle injected the ink into my skin at the top of my sternum (breast bone). These dots will be with me forever. To someone who doesn't know, they might look like freckles. To me, I am now "marked" forever.

The radiation technicians who completed the markings were informative about the process of radiation. The markings (tattoos) took about half an hour to complete. My biggest challenge was trying to get my right arm over my head because this position exposed my underarm and right side of my chest to the radiation machine. I had very good range of arm motion before the sepsis; however, that range of motion was now lost. It hurt to stretch my arm over my head, but I did it.

On April 6th, Kevin brought me to the radiation clinic for my first treatment. I was nervous because I didn't know what to expect. When I went to reception, I was given a list of my appointments for the week. Kevin had to stay in the general waiting room and was not allowed to wait in the lobby beside the radiation equipment to provide patients with some privacy as we all wore patient gowns. There were only a couple of people waiting in the lobby for the radiation machine. No one really talked much. In fact, I found it much quieter in this treatment area than the chemo area; many people talked in the chemo area, possible related to a greater sense of normalcy related to wearing street clothing.

Before each of my thirty treatments, the technicians asked my name, date of birth and something else (perhaps my address) just to make sure I was the right person. That is probably a good habit to have in their business because I wouldn't want to get the wrong dose of radiation.

The first procedure took extra time because the technicians needed to arrange my position prior to the treatment. I lay down on the radiation table and put my arm in a special contraption so it couldn't move. The technicians lined up my hips according to the tattooed dots in a process resembling that of an airplane coming toward the runway when landing, pull here, turn there. My body was very stiff because I was scared. After I was "lined up," the technicians left the room to go behind a lead shield that protects them from exposure to radiation. If necessary, I could talk to the technicians through an intercom.

Each day, I had four sequential doses of radiation. The first two doses of radiation to the main area of my right chest and side area also involved the use of a bolus cloth, which was made of a special material that intensified the dose of radiation to my skin. I mentally prepared for the first dose, remembering Kate's advice to recite "the Lord is my Shepherd" to help calm myself; I began mentally reciting the words as the noise from the machine started; it was like the noise out of a science fiction show. Each dose of radiation lasted about ten to fifteen seconds. After the right side of my breast area was done, the technician moved the bolus cloth towards my sternum. The noise started again, and once again I recited the twenty-third Psalm from the beginning. Another ten to fifteen seconds passed and the second dose was over. The technicians removed the bolus cloth and ensured I was still lined up according to the tattoos before the third dose of radiation occurred from under the radiation table. The machine slowly turned around and the noise started again; I recited the psalm again. Another ten to fifteen seconds passed. Finally, the fourth dose began at the top of my lung and armpit (or at least this is where I think it started). The first session was over, and I climbed off the radiation table. I was surprised that the treatment didn't hurt. The whole session took about thirty minutes, but the technicians told me my next session would be shorter. This radiation routine happened four times the first week because radiation was not scheduled on Good Friday or Easter Monday.

Every week I attended Dr. Pereira's clinic to review my progress and provide any ongoing assistance. The first week was a cinch because I adjusted easily to the routine. First, I applied aloe vera gel to cool my skin and prevent burning, followed by moisturizing cream. During the first week of treatment, my skin turned pink after radiation but returned to its regular colour within thirty minutes. By the end of the second week, I noticed that my skin was getting itchy, and by the end of the third week (the thirteenth treatment), my skin was really itchy. The doctor gave me a steroid cream to help with the itching that was to be applied sparingly. I really wanted to scratch my skin overtly but I didn't. Instead I relieved the itching by thoroughly rubbing in the cream. To my surprise, this was a big mistake. I rationalized as a nurse, "Doesn't rubbing in the cream into the skin help it get absorbed by the tissue better?" Apparently, this is not so! The radiology nurse told me, in a rather condescending manner, that rubbing in the cream further damages the skin that is already in trouble. My skin was now red all the time. Around the seventh treatment, my skin started blistering. I saw Dr. Pereira and, to my relief, he said the bolus cloth could come off.

At the end of April, I had a follow-up appointment with Dr. Potvin, my chemo oncologist. She reviewed the biopsy results and told me that as far as she was concerned, I was cancer free. I wondered, *Is this my Easter miracle?* I told her I was struggling to see myself surviving and having a future.

In response, she described other women whom she told were cancer free. They were so worried about the return of the cancer that they did not have any quality of life. Their lives were frozen in "cancer time." I could really identify with these women, but I did not want to share their fate so I decided to try and internalize this advice. *I was the doubting Thomas.* I vowed to subdue my fear. That afternoon, I met Leonie on her way home from school and told her that Dr. Potvin had said I was "cancer free." Then I promptly asked her if she would stop visualizing me dying every day. We both laughed and she agreed. Leonie stopped "killing me" every day after that. Coincidentally, her headaches and stomach aches virtually disappeared after that day. What a relief not to have to deal with that emotional pain every day.

School, however, was much more difficult to fix. Leonie was fearful at school, and she continued to miss about half of her school time due to illness. Leonie asked every day if she could be home schooled. Therefore, I taught her a mantra, hoping it would help her to relax and feel safe:

I am safe in Guatemala
I am safe with Mom and Dad and even Eliza too.
I am safe with my friends Catie, Emily and Amy.
I am safe at school with Ms. M. (her teacher).
I can be happy because it makes my mom happy.

Leonie would try to repeat it to help calm herself. Sometimes it worked, but sometimes her fearfulness and anxiety were too much to be calmed by the mantra.

I also arranged for Leonie to experience some counselling. The cancer clinic told me they didn't have services for children and I thought that this was a terrible shame. I called Leonie's elementary school and made arrangements for Leonie to see the school counsellor, Mr. H., so she could talk to him about how she was feeling. This process went very slowly. I also arranged for my friend Mary, who is a master's prepared social worker with a specialty in children's therapy, to talk with Leonie so that Leonie could hopefully share her fears. Leonie preferred these visits when they went out for ice cream. Mary and Leonie only met a couple of times because I think Leonie wanted to move on after she believed that I was going to live.

Kevin and I continued to struggle over my need for him to take over the management of our home, instead of relying on me to co-ordinate everything. I knew that he possessed the necessary skills, but he was becoming more stressed and feeling the pressure to work even harder at his job. He would always provide the excuse "I'm trying my best." His "best," however, wasn't reducing my burden. At home, he would view success as tasks completed rather than from the perspective of relationship and values. We would talk about something needing to be changed; he would agree and then nothing would change. I felt guilty asking for more and angry that I was so vulnerable having to almost to beg for change. It was so draining, and I now knew that this stage had to end. I asked him to go back to the counsellor and try and get some more insight into the problem. I needed him to take charge of his development and to understand his emotions and how they affect the family. It was time for the girls to do chores and to be on time without him getting frustrated with them. I was afraid that all the girls would remember was the frustration and not see they weren't being responsible for themselves.

The Friday before Mother's Day, Kevin and I went out to a plant nursery to buy blossoming trees or bushes to give to our friends who had driven me to radiation every week. My skin was quite blistered and sore, so I walked holding my clothes away from my body. There were many beautiful blossoming trees everywhere, but their beauty could not reduce my pain. After about thirty minutes of looking around, I asked Kevin if we could leave. When I got home, the blisters had burst and the fluid had leaked onto my clothes. When I took my clothes off, my skin came off with my shirt. The skin was so raw underneath that it wept and bled. My eyes also leaked; I cried like a river. My skin was so sore; it hurt all day and all night. It even hurt to breathe. I spent the weekend in bed because it hurt to move. Kevin returned by himself to purchase the bushes we selected.

Now, I thought, Mother's Day was going to be even worse than ever because I would be in pronounced physical pain in addition to the regular emotional pain I experienced every year, since my mother had died on Mother's Day when I was five years old. This Mother's Day I vowed that if I made it another year, I would make every Mother's Day in the future much nicer for myself and my family.

After Mother's Day, my radiation burn felt torturous. It hurt to bend over; I walked hunched over because I couldn't stand to have anything, such as clothing, touch my skin. The burn had now gone all the way through to the back of my shoulder blade. It hurt a lot on my chest below the incision line. Every day, I had to use an antibiotic cream that is frequently used for burn patients to prevent infection in the open areas of skin. In fact, the care of my skin took about two hours each day. Dr. Pereira told me to use Epsom salts to soothe the open areas and then to use a hair dryer to dry the skin before I put on the antibiotic cream. Drying the skin with a hair dryer actually allowed the cream to adhere to my skin rather than slide off. It hurt a lot to care for my skin, and I cried a lot.

There are two individual patients' stories I would like to relate now because they are so memorable to me. I only met one other patient who appeared to have a radiation burn more severe than mine. One day as I was checking in at the reception desk of the radiation clinic, I noticed her skin at the top of her blouse. I could see she also had a pretty severe radiation burn. I said to her that she was the only person I had met so far who seemed to have a radiation burn that seemed worse than mine. She then showed me her skin, and I could see her radiation burn was actually worse than mine. The scab on her skin was very crusty and about one half inch thick. She told me she had fainted from pain that morning cleaning her skin. I don't know if anyone told her about cleaning her skin with Epsom salts and about debriding the scar (not letting the scab accumulate). What a hard world it is for people who don't know these things.

The second woman I met during radiation had stage four breast cancer for fifteen years. She told me she had received chemo or radiation most of the time during that period. Even though her doctors thought she would die, she clearly didn't. The most amazing part was she seemed very optimistic about her future: chemo and radiation were just normal parts of her life.

I think that both these women knew what it was like to be on the cross at Golgotha. The woman who had treatment for fifteen years was like the prisoner who, even in her suffering, felt privileged to be alive. The woman with the radiation burn was so distraught, she felt abandoned in her suffering. She had even fainted from the pain.

About half way through my treatment, I had another interesting experience. There were only a couple of radiation machines that can do advanced treatments, and I needed one of them. When my machine became overbooked, I was transferred to another section of the radiation clinic. It turned out the other machine was almost solely used for men with prostate cancer. It seemed to me that I was the first woman scheduled to use that machine. We had quite polite conversation while I sat in my patient shirt and the prostate men sat in their pyjama bottoms. Sitting there seemed surreal, like we were in another world.

My second last week of treatment, I saw Dr. Pereira. He marked me for my last five treatments. These last five treatments focused on the skin around the incision line in order to reduce the risk of the cancer returning. Apparently, cancer cells can "hide" in the skin. Dr. Pereira drew the markings with a black magic marker on clear plastic that looked like the plastic that goes on an overhead machine. The markings resembled the shape of a huge peanut. The next week when I went for the treatments, the technicians placed a metal template on the machine exactly like the peanut drawing and I did not have to put my arm over my head anymore—this was a very small mercy. Nevertheless, around the twenty-sixth day, my skin was so burnt the technicians asked whether I wanted to go through with the treatment or postpone my treatment a few days. I thought the waiting would only make things worse. I had noticed a very small improvement in some of the areas where the treatment had been completed, so I proceeded with the treatment.

One day near the end of my treatments, I was walking up the stairs at the cancer clinic and I got a terrible pain down my right leg. Later that night, my leg felt numb. I felt very afraid, not knowing if something serious was occurring, so I called the on-call doctors at the cancer clinic. They didn't have any explanation for the numbness and pain. That night, I took a sedative to calm myself and went to bed. Walking was very painful, and now I couldn't bend over to even tie my shoe—how humbling. I wondered if the pain was because of bone cancer, so I went to my family doctor. Dr. Kumar thought I had sciatica (pain in my back and right leg). By this time I thought that radiation was really torture. In addition to the sciatica that continued for the next two months, I now felt the extreme fatigue commonly associated with radiation. The fatigue was not predictable and could hit at any time or any place. Dr. Pereira told me most people think that radiation is the easiest part of the treatment. For me, sepsis was the worst part, closely followed by radiation.

Jesus had trouble walking with his cross. He was fatigued and his strength was sapped. Someone carried his cross. I also was fatigued and had trouble walking. I felt completely broken. Do people carry invisible crosses?

During my visits with Dr. Pereira, I found out that 75 percent of my breast had been cancerous. I also found out there was an irregular spot that showed up on my sternum during the bone scan. It wasn't over activity, representing bone cancer; it was under activity (meaning that area of my sternum was under functioning) and the doctors were not sure why that was occurring. The radiologist suggested the bone scan should be repeated in six months. Dr. Pereira said there really was no sense in repeating the bone scan right now because there would be under activity in my ribs and sternum as a side effect of the radiation. Dr. Pereira said he would review the results of the bone scan at my next appointment in the fall.

The kindest part of radiation therapy came from the people who drove me to the cancer clinic each day. I had organized a roster so different people drove me each day while Kevin drove on the days when I had a doctor's appointment. The sympathy I felt from my drivers when my skin deteriorated told me how much I was loved.

The women at our church also called after hearing of my plight and arranged to deliver some meals to our family. I was so grateful. Only one person didn't really understand our need for nutritious home-cooked meals and gave us $100 to go out for food, to eat in a restaurant. We donated this money to the church.

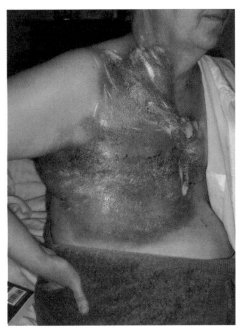

A picture of the radiation burn just after the radiation treatment was completed. The silver is the result of the antibiotic burn cream. You can see some healing above and below the incision. The open areas in the skin were closing. The deep red patches around the incision line were still weeping and bleeding, but not as bad as earlier. In hindsight, I am glad I did not take a picture of the wound completely bleeding, with the skin entirely traumatized. I want to forget that point in my life.

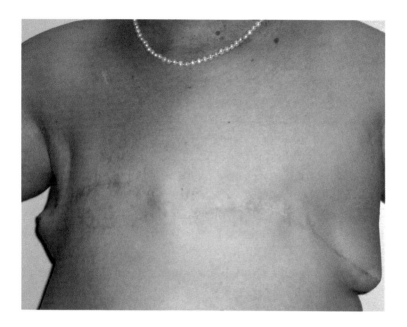

One year later, my skin is returning to its normal colour. You can see some spider veins near the incision on the right side. You have to be very close to see the radiation tattoos. You can really see the miracle of healing when you compare the pictures of the radiation burn to my skin right now. I will probably always have the skin flaps to the side of the chest where the surgical drains were inserted.

At the end of my thirty radiation treatments, I ordered an ice cream cake for the staff in radiation to say thanks. Ice cream seemed symbolic since it is the opposite of radiation: cold takes away the heat. I brought the cake in twenty minutes early, before my appointment, and I had pre-arranged for the staff to bring in a knife to cut the cake since I didn't think it would be a good idea to register for the clinic with a big knife in my bag. Then a technician came and said, "I can take you right now if you are ready." By the time I came out of my treatment room, the cake had been all distributed and the staff were smiling. Now that is both good will and efficiency!

Kevin and I also gave lovely flowering bushes to our friends who had helped drive me to the clinic. We had a party, and Kate came to our house and blessed all of the bushes and gave thanks to God for everyone who had helped me get through my treatment. Then we had dessert together. I hoped I would see each of the bushes bloom the following year.

Prayer was now about the only thing I could do to help others. I also learned to listen better to other people's troubles without owning their problems. Sometimes I would give advice, but not very often. I would pray for them afterwards, because I knew that was all I could really do. I do know that one of my prayers was answered. My sister moved back to London, Ontario, from Michigan in May, 2009. What a relief! I could see her and not have to worry constantly that something bad would happen to her and I couldn't be there to help.

Reflections:

- I wonder if my skin had such a severe reaction to the radiation because my body was wearing down after the chemo, surgery and sepsis.
- Patients need to know not to rub the steroid cream into the skin.
- The cumulative effect of radiation is severe with unpredictable fatigue.
- The kindness of receiving home-made nutritious meals really helped us.
- It is right to give thanks and praise. The ice cream cake and flowering bushes made a difference to the people who helped us.
- Even though the treatment did end, the suffering didn't.
- I promise to treasure Mother's Day for myself and for my family forever.

Chapter 5

Easter Saturday: Hormone Therapy

Even though hormones are hidden in the body, you can see their effects. Jesus' body was hidden in the tomb. We don't really know what happened to Jesus on Easter Saturday. He was probably cared for by hidden angels. May my medications to suppress estrogen act like these hidden angels.

Because my tumour was sensitive to estrogen (meaning the tumour needed estrogen to grow), Dr. Potvin discussed hormone therapy with me in April. I would be safer (meaning less chance of the cancer returning) with lower levels of estrogen in my body. Dr. Potvin initially prescribed Tamoxifen in April because I was terrified that the cancer would return due to the increased number of lymph nodes that were positive for cancer. Apparently Tamoxifen is a medication that blocks the effect of estrogen in the breast. Nevertheless, Dr. Potvin wanted me to be on Femara that suppresses estrogen (reduces the estrogen levels throughout the body). This drug is a fertility drug used in pre-menopausal women and, ironically, an estrogen suppressant in post-menopausal women. Since I had not had a menstrual period since after my first chemo treatments, Dr. Potvin did not want to start me on the estrogen suppressant until she was confidant I was in menopause and not just in chemo-induced menopause.

I was very fortunate that I was not plagued with hot flashes as a side effect of Tamoxifen. My current hot flashes were never as bad as the literal trial by fire I had experienced when the chemo put me into menopause over a weekend during the previous October (at the beginning of my chemo). Now when the hot flashes occurred, usually unexpectedly, I would just loosen my clothing and wait them out. They would pass in about five minutes. I didn't like being on Tamoxifen because I was worried about another possible side effect: blood clots in my legs. When do you suppose I will have exhausted all of my worries?

In June, 2009, I began attending a special clinic with both Dr. Potvin and Dr. Powers (a reproductive endocrinologist). The first step in beginning to change my medication to the estrogen suppressant was to check the hormone levels in my blood to see if they were low, indicating menopause. The blood work indicated I had lower estrogen levels, but the only way to be sure was to monitor my progress over time. Dr. Powers completed an internal ultrasound to measure the ovaries to see if they were "silent" (not producing estrogen) and check for any irregular masses. My uterine lining was getting thinner, another good sign that I was in menopause. The ultrasound also showed no extra fluid (a potential sign of ovarian cancer).

At the initial visit, Dr. Powers said some of the most comforting words I have ever heard. He told me his plan was to help me be around so I could be a grandmother. When I met him, I thought that I recognized Dr. Powers and he me. He said, "Have we met before?" and I said, "Oh yes. I was at the fertility clinic here ten years ago when I had five miscarriages. You did an emergency surgery when I was hemorrhaging and had an infection." I smiled and said, "At least the next time I see you, you won't be doing an emergency D & C on me." He gave me a hug.

I began taking the estrogen suppressant drug June 2nd, 2009. Within days of taking the estrogen suppressant, my head felt really "spaced out" and I felt a little dizzy. After a couple of days of these symptoms, I remembered, that when I was on a fertility drug ten years earlier, the nurse had suggested I take the drug at night and sleep through some of the side effects, and this approach reduced the dizziness and the sleepiness at bedtime. The estrogen suppressant was not, however, a good fit with the sedative (the anti-anxiety drug) that I was taking most nights to sleep. It took me almost two weeks to wean myself off the sedative.

I soon rediscovered that the stereotype about women on fertility drugs was true in my case. I was often emotionally volatile and irrational. When I was frustrated, mad or sad, I was no longer able to refrain from holding back my emotions and they just came pouring out. This change in my personality was perhaps the biggest transition my family faced; they saw the real me when I was upset, and it didn't look or feel pretty. It was very obvious now that I was frustrated with our family life. I wondered if I would ever be able to reduce the stress and frustration levels. I knew our family coping mechanisms needed to change if I was going to get some quality of life. It was daunting to know I could be so emotionally out of control for the five years that I would be on the drug. I am very grateful to have the opportunity to take this drug because I know it will improve my chances of survival; I was just lamenting that I may feel emotionally out of control for five years.

Reflections:

- Hormones have a big effect on your self-image and recovery.
- There is no more potent truth serum than a fertility drug.
- Hearing Dr. Powers tell me he is going to help me become a grandmother may be the sweetest words I have ever heard.
- Life circles: I was on a fertility drug ten years ago to try and create another life. Now I was on a fertility drug to try and save my life.

Chapter 6

Adversity Story
Karen Adamson

Pat, my childhood friend of forty years, was diagnosed with stage three breast cancer last September—almost one year ago today. She and I were inseparable as children growing up in small-town Ontario. There really were four of us in our group: Pat, Cathy, Vicki and me, who bonded as best friends throughout elementary and secondary school. Pat, Cathy and Vicki ameliorated my escape from childhood unhappiness. My mother suffered from depression, which was undiagnosed and untreated at that time; her unpredictable behaviour caused me much grief and suffering. Pat's mother died from pancreatic cancer when she was five years old, thereby adding to Pat's feelings of abandonment that began when her father abandoned the family a few years before her mother died. We three girls became Pat's surrogate family, helping to fill the empty space left by the loss of her parents. You may find it surprising to learn that Pat was the clown of our little group. She kept us all laughing and, as a result, taught us to cope with adversity through humour.

After secondary school graduation, we all went our separate ways in order to shape our future lives and careers and lost close touch with one another for a while. I moved to

Toronto to live and study, Pat decided to settle in London, Ontario, Vicki left for Alberta, never to return to Ontario, and Cathy chose to remain in our small town.

Pat and I did see each other a few times a year during our twenties, became close again in our thirties, and then for a time we lost touch completely. Ten years went by, during which Pat had two children, worked in several high-level, demanding jobs and completed her PhD in sociology. I spent that time going through the break up of a long-term relationship and battling depression.

I reunited with my future husband but Pat and I continued to drift further and further apart. On the outside, we appeared to be busy, fulfilled and accomplished—hadn't Pat and I persevered and triumphed? All the same, we both suffered from profound feelings of loneliness. It took more life experience and self-reflection on both our parts for us to realize that our lives felt empty without our friendship—we missed the loving, close bond that we used to enjoy and the active role we played in each other's lives.

You may be wondering why I have recounted this past history. I am convinced that our past history is a significant part of my life journey and of Pat's life journey, and it continues to play a vital role in our friendship.

One year before our fiftieth birthdays, Pat and I reconnected, vowing to never again let our friendship wane. For two years, our friendship thrived, both of us celebrating and strengthening our relationship. Then Pat learned that she had stage three breast cancer; her prognosis was dismal and uncertain. In any event, she was told that her treatment would be extensive, arduous and painful. Because she characterized the heart and strength of her family (as many women do), her husband and children found it extremely difficult to cope with her illness.

Pat's life-threatening cancer constituted a crossroads for me. I knew that whatever path I chose to take would impact me for the rest of my life. Could I face the fact that she may be taken out of my life permanently at a time when we had never been closer, and could I cope with seeing her go through a gruelling, year-long treatment process that was not guaranteed to provide a cure, would negatively impact her quality of life, and possibly shorten the time she had left to live? Some of Pat's loved ones could not deal with these pressures and chose to extricate themselves from her illness and her struggle to overcome it. Having always pondered what I would do in a situation that embodies one of my worst fears—facing my own death or that of a dearly loved friend or family member— I found myself meeting this situation head on. I agonized over my doubts—would I be strong enough to provide for the needs of my dying loved one—or would I wimp out and find an excuse to position myself on the periphery, allowing others to step in and give the vital help that she required?

In the end my choice became clear. I knew that it would be far more excruciatingly painful for me to stand by the sidelines, thereby extricating myself from Pat's life, than it would be to join wholeheartedly in her struggle to defeat this devastating cancer. It turned out to be almost effortless for me to put myself in Pat's place because of our shared history and our committed bond—it felt to me as if I had been diagnosed with cancer. At the same time, there no doubt in my mind that if our positions were reversed, Pat would be there for me. Despite knowing that the struggle could demand more than I am capable of giving, I chose to follow that path with heart.

Now that the year of treatment is over and Pat has been told that she is cancer free, I can admit that the journey was far harder than I ever imagined. When the chemotherapy sapped her strength, removed all the hair from her body, and made her favourite foods taste like acid, I fought to keep my faith that she was going to beat cancer and live. And when radiation therapy burned her skin so badly she could not wear clothes without severe pain, it took all my inner strength to remain positive and act as if her skin was not utterly ravaged by radiation burns. Most of all, I was forced to tackle my deep-seated fear that she would die and leave me all alone, all the while believing it was necessary to hide my inner struggle from Pat and her family.

Although Pat and I know that medically speaking she is cancer free, it will take time for us to accept it, as Pat says, on a soul level. She tells me that she can only pray for one more year of life right now, but in a year or so she might be able to ask the Divine Presence for two or three more years. It was just the other day that she confided that her anger about growing up without a mother fuels her resolve to not only survive, but to completely eradicate her cancer. She declared, "I am damned determined that my girls will not grow up without a mother like I did." The willpower, courage and utter lack of self-pity that Pat showed during this past year serve as a living example of grace and strength for her girls and for me. She is my beloved hero.

Adversity Story Poem

We were childhood friends, best friends; small town angst fuelled our unhappiness, our desire to spread our wings and leave.

Taking our leave alone, fearing abandonment and loneliness, despite the courage to begin anew.

We joined surrogate families in going our separate ways, living our lives with an intensity that turned into accomplishment and triumph, despite occasional depression.

Profound emptiness surfaced in mid-life reflection; our life journeys were at a crossroads—we were living on the periphery of feeling—not thriving, nor suffering.

Subsisting on the sidelines saps strength, subjugates joy, triggers agonizing doubts.

Painful diagnosis showed the way to reconnection, reattachment—a resolve to take the path with heart.

Once again she was my devoted friend and my hero.

What is a hero?

One who lives comfortably with a full expression of feeling without self-pity, full of grace and courage.

Chapter 7

The Peaceable Kingdom
Kevin Webb

There is a passage in Isaiah 11:6 of the Bible (KJV) that states, *"The wolf also shall dwell with the lamb, and the leopard shall lie down with the kid; and the calf and the young lion and the fatling together; and a little child shall lead them."*

I have always interpreted this passage literally as everyone and everything living in a world without conflict. That has now changed. The challenges that we, as a family, faced with my wife's breast cancer coupled with the increased stresses of my job have caused me to interpret this passage at a much deeper and personal level.

In many ways it is ironic that the "Peaceable Kingdom" was my next cross stitch project during our family's experience of breast cancer. Counted cross stitch is a hobby that I started in 1981, almost thirty years ago. I used to read voraciously, and if I had a good book I wouldn't stop reading until it was completed or I was too tired to read anymore, which can be a problem. I started cross stitch because you could put it down at any time. I found its repetitiveness very relaxing. I liked the idea of creating something out of an empty canvas. So I replaced reading (not completely) with cross stitch and proceeded to do it until I was too tired to do it anymore. Nothing really changed, since, as this experience taught me, I can have an obsessive personality. I don't like to quit!

I have completed more than thirty cross stitch pictures over the past thirty years with each one becoming more and more elaborate. When I was completing my last picture, Da Vinci's Last Supper, which we were donating to our church, Pat bemoaned the fact that I had never done a picture just for her. "Okay," I said, "What do you want?" She said she had always loved the concept of the Peaceable Kingdom and could I find such a cross stitch? We searched and found one online and ordered the pattern book.

It arrived in December 2007, and I was taken aback. It was a picture of a painting done by Thomas Hicks in 1834. It was beautiful. It was also the largest and most complicated cross stitch that I had ever seen. There were over 100 colours, all of them blended (two different colours of embroidery floss), and the total stitch count approached 150,000! To put this in perspective, Da Vinci's Last Supper had approximately 45,000 stitches and took me two years to complete. The Last Supper, however, had fewer colours and none of them were blended. I predicted that this project could take me up to ten years to complete.

I began the cross stitch in January 2008, which was the time when Pat began noticing that her breast was sore. Little did I know at that time the challenges that lay ahead. My clearest recollections of that spring and summer were of Pat being worried and tired. Me, the "short-term optimist" believed the health system that said it was mastitis and it was not serious. I worked diligently on the new cross stitch. I was tracking my progress on this project by counting the number of stitches on each of the forty-four pages in the pattern book (3,564 per page) and how long it took to com-plete each page, sort of like a journal. *By July 20, 2008, I had completed four pages (14,466 stitches)* . My obsessive-ness with a new project is very evident. Given the shock to the family with Pat's cancer, it is not surprising that it took me until December 20, 2008 to complete the next page.

I clearly remember the day when Pat was diagnosed with breast cancer. It was August 28, 2008. Our brand new (expensive) sunroom was being completed, and Pat's nephew Mike was helping me (actually I was helping him because I am not very handy) construct a new modular shed. I had taken Pat to St. Joe's hospital for a mammo-gram. Pat said she would call when she needed to be picked up. Since I was in the backyard with Mike, I couldn't hear the phone. I had asked Eliza and Leonie, our daughters, to listen for the phone and to let me know if it was Mom. Needless to say, the phone rang, I didn't hear it, and the girls didn't pick it up! Fortunately Pat remembered Mike's cell phone number and called him.

As I drove the ten minutes to pick up Pat, I was wor-ried because she had sounded both angry and scared on the phone. I apologized when I picked her up, and all she could say was that she had "flunked" the tests. "What does that mean," I asked? "It's cancer!" I still didn't fully comprehend the import of what she said, but I knew cancer was potentially fatal although most of them are now very treatable. Again I was the short-term optimist and felt she would be fine. *I had completed 15,000 stitches on my cross stitch!*

Pat and I met in 1987 at church. While I love Pat, our love has been based more upon our friendship and mutual respect. We never "fell in love" but drifted into it as we spent more and more time together. We decided to buy a house together, not out of love, but as a business proposition. We were friends at the time (1989) and both wanted to settle down in a house. The thought was that we would own the house for a few years, sell it and then go our separate ways. But something happened between making that decision and actually buying the house in May 1990. We found that we enjoyed being in each other's company. We felt like family. In June, 1990, our minister's wife, Rose, whom we dearly loved, was diagnosed with ovarian cancer. Pat started to cry when we found out and said tearfully, "Life is too short, do you want to get married?" We decided to get married, and over the years, the love did come, not as an epiphany, but slowly and quietly. We had our "discussions" and frustrations as in any relationship, but our friendship never waned.

Pat and I were married on September 15, 1990. One of the reasons we chose that date was that nothing would interfere with our anniversaries. For ten years, we would go to Mackinac Island (located in Michigan) for a few days around our anniversary. It was always wonderful. Since the island doesn't allow private vehicles, the only way to get around on the island is to walk, bicycle or hire a horse-drawn taxi. We found the perfect place to stay— Mission Point Resort, because it was large enough to have a lounge and large common areas where you could relax and read. Since the weather tended to be unpredictable on the island during September, this was a tremendous benefit during rainy days. One of our favourite activities was walking around the island (eight miles) and up to Fort Holmes, which looked down on Fort Mackinac, the town and the straits. A few days on the island felt like a week of peaceful respite.

It has been at least ten years since we have gone to Mackinac Island for our anniversary. I am the Chief Administrative Officer for an international development organization, and since 2000, I have been required to attend a national conference each September and give at least one presentation. This conference usually occurred the week of our anniversary. In 2008, the annual conference was in Victoria, British Columbia. Now, we were "not only" not going on vacation, but I had to leave home when then was a family crisis.

With Pat's diagnosis confirmed on September 2nd by the surgeon, Dr. Holiday, I was in conflict over whether I should stay home or go to Victoria. This conference was going to be a busy time for me because not only did I have to give a presentation but I was also to participate in a key breakout meeting to discuss the new direction being taken by our organization. By August 28th, all of the travel plans were in place. I had the plane tickets and my hotel reservations. Pat and I discussed it, and since her oncology appointment was not until September 15th (another irony as it is our anniversary) and I was returning late on September 14th, she felt it was okay for me to go. In hindsight, which is always "20/20," I should probably have stayed home and helped support Pat and the girls. It is amazing that at the time you feel that there isn't a choice, but then afterwards you realize that there was a choice and perhaps you were simply not as flexible as you should have been. My obsessiveness was showing again.

I have never considered myself as a "Pollyanna," always seeing the positives, always knowing things will work out for the best, but I never had a doubt that Pat would win the battle with breast cancer. I believe this helped her because while she was contemplating her imminent death, I was thinking about our life after we had beat cancer. The downside of this attitude is that I probably didn't fully understand how close she actually came to having the cancer metastasize to other areas of her body. Pat has mentioned to me several times that she was probably only a month or so away from it spreading to the rest of her body if she hadn't started getting treatment immediately.

I returned home from Victoria after a very long day just after midnight on September 15th. I managed to get a few hours of sleep before we were off to the cancer clinic and the initial consult with the oncologist, Dr. Potvin. She was very direct in saying that, yes, it was cancer and that it was "locally advanced breast cancer." She also said that it was completely treatable but that Pat would have a very difficult year.

Pat has detailed her story in the other chapters of this book, so I will not reiterate it here but focus on my own emotional development during this very stressful time. In order to help with the context of our family's crisis during Pat's treatment and recovery from breast cancer, I have included some personal information from my childhood and my relationship with my family.

I was born in England, and my family emigrated to Canada when I was ten years old. For years I harboured a resentment and anger that I was the cause for the uprooting of everything we knew and loved. Of course, I realize now that this was just the imaginings of a sensitive ten-year-old boy. But when we came to Canada, there was a change in the relationship between my parents and me. They, as most first generation immigrants do, held to the old ways, which were fortunately not too different than the Canadian ways. However, it was difficult for me to make friends as I was both shy and quiet and dressed differently. In England, school children wore uniforms, and my mother would insist that I be well dressed for school and have a haircut (when everyone else had longer hair in the later 1960s), which made me a bit of a pariah with my peers.

I can't say that my childhood family was ever really emotionally close. Feelings were never discussed. It was always assumed that you were loved, with no outward expressions of love. Being the oldest of three siblings, I was expected to "set the example" of good behaviour. I became a withdrawn teenager, quiet, insecure and emotionally distant. I developed a stutter when I spoke.

During my adult years, I would often withdraw when I encountered highly emotional situations. I would physically be unable to speak! It was as though I had physically lost the ability to talk. I recall a time when Pat was very upset with me a couple of years after we were married. I withdrew into my shell, and understandably she became even more upset. When we returned home, she went crying to our bedroom and I sat on the couch very angry with myself. One of the most difficult things I have ever done was to then go upstairs and say sorry. This represented one of the most dramatic changes in my life because since then, I have found it easier to discuss my feelings while under emotional stress.

Having your own family can be excellent therapy because attachment and honesty are at the heart of the familial relationship. Prior to Pat's cancer, I believed I was a good parent and husband. I cooked, cleaned, did the groceries, took the children to their various activities, told them I loved them, etc. While this was true to an extent, I was really only there physically. I was not as emotionally attached as I should have been. This was quite evident as Eliza became a preteen and then a teenager. We would squabble all the time, usually over small insignificant things that only seemed important in the heat of the argument. Pat felt like she had three children in the house, and I felt like no one was on my side. Upon reflection, I was probably living out my teenage anger towards my parents and siblings during this time.

As you can see from these past couple of paragraphs, I had my personal "demons" that I needed to understand and exorcise. This is where the concept of the Peaceable Kingdom becomes relevant. As I indicated at the beginning of this chapter, the "literal" interpretation is living in a world without conflict. However, as I dealt with the challenges caused by the introduction of cancer into the family, the Peaceable Kingdom took on a personal and deeper meaning. It became my personal search for inner peace and understanding, to help me become a better parent, husband and friend.

Change is always difficult because it means replacing something that is known, understandable and comfortable with something that is unknown, not immediately understandable and often uncomfortable, at least in the short term. For many of us, it feels like the change is due to us having done something wrong. Change is also easier if you are the one directing the change. For the past few years at work, change has been the predominant theme, as we adapted to a new international development paradigm of program management. In my job, I was required to develop and implement the new protocols and procedures. However, changing "me" was different. My insecurities and feelings of inadequacy again came to the forefront. I became passive and more withdrawn. I was stressed, without fully understanding that I was stressed. I literally withdrew into "the cave" every evening, which in this case was the family room in the basement. I became more obsessive with my cross-stitch, which I often did when I watched television. I started and completed a different picture as a Christmas gift for Mike and Michelle, Pat's nephew and niece, and their young daughter, Livvy (Olivia). The Peaceable Kingdom cross stitch picture continually beckoned me like a siren. *By December 28, 2008, I had completed 17,820 cross stitches.*

However, during the day I felt that I was very engaged in supporting Pat. I was taking Pat to all of her chemotherapy appointments, and this quickly developed into a routine. I would drop her off at the door, find a parking spot, join her in the clinic and wait to be called. In the pre-chemo meetings, I would take notes because Pat was starting to have difficulty remembering details (chemo brain). Once the appointment was finished, I would drive Pat home and we would either spend a few minutes talking about the appointment or I would head off to work. My job during this period was very busy and stressful as I was responsible for submitting the program funding proposal to the federal government. Also, there was a three-day board meeting at the end of October followed by a trip to Ottawa in early November.

By 8:00 p.m., I felt I had done "my bit" and retired to the basement. However, the evening wasn't done because this was when the girls would seek comfort and guidance.

Leonie was decompensating and didn't want to be separated from her mom. Eliza redirected all of her energies into school. This was a good thing, but she often brought home her frustrations about the "injustices inflicted upon her by unfeeling teachers or other students." Neither Eliza nor Leonie had a lot of patience for each other. Since I was "absent," they went to Pat. Petty jealousies raged around how much time each other was spending with Mom.

Pat became more frustrated and angry with me, accusing me of not wanting to be around her or the girls. "Don't you like us anymore?" She felt that I put a higher priority on work than the needs of the family. It was difficult to explain my actions since they were so deep rooted that the reasons were lost in the deep-seated memories of my past. When confronted by Pat, I only withdrew even more and became visibly depressed. Pat would give up because she was so exhausted and would say, "Let's try again tomorrow."

I felt bad but didn't know how to break the cycle. At Pat's recommendation, I started going to counselling at the cancer clinic. The first few sessions were pretty good, and I believe that I did make progress. In the late evenings, I would come upstairs and be with Pat, so that she had an opportunity to discuss her day. My presence also seemed to reduce the time the girls wanted to spend with Mom.

At around this time, Pat and the girls all complained about my snoring. Pat was having trouble sleeping with the snoring, and she was getting more and more tired. Leonie said her walls shook. Even though this was a bit of an exaggeration, I agreed to move out of the bedroom into the family room in the basement. We rearranged some of the furniture to provide me with a bed, and it seemed to work.

My sessions with the counsellor were having a positive effect on me. They gave me a chance to ventilate my feelings in a safe environment, and this helped keep my stress level down. In turn, this enabled me to think more clearly about my relationship with Eliza and gain a greater understanding of how I was reliving my dysfunctional adolescence with her. However, the progress began to stall and Pat suggested that she also attend one of the counselling sessions. I agreed, and we both attended the one scheduled for November. Pat had an epiphany during this session, because for the first time she understood that I need to feel uncomfortable before I could change my "personal paradigm." I needed to suffer first to be able to make the change. Pat had always sought to minimize my suffering. Whenever we had a disagreement and I felt bad afterwards, she would attempt to comfort me—to take away the suffering. Her logic was that she had suffered as a child and didn't want others to suffer. But all this did was perpetuate the cycle without any change on my part. With this realization, she promised to let me suffer during and after a disagreement to see if my behaviour did actually change. Sometimes you do get what you ask for! With this understanding, change did come from my suffering—not immediately but gradually over the next several months.

I realized that I was reacting to Eliza's anxieties as though they were directed against me. I was defensive and always having my feelings bruised. Once I understood that she was "railing against the world" and I was just a convenient target, I stopped taking it so personally. Life improved dramatically, and Eliza actually started settling down when I didn't argue or debate as much with her.

Helping Leonie was more difficult because she was

afraid of losing her mom, not her dad. Leonie fell in love with me at "first sight" when we first met her in Guatemala in 2001. Even though she adored me and was very quick to defend my every action, she did not come to me when she was upset. She would only go to Pat. She decompensated if I became frustrated with her. Then she would go and tell Pat how I had hurt her and been "unfair." It took me a long time to learn to listen to both of the girls feelings, without interrupting and without giving advice, unless they asked for it.

The disagreements with Pat began to decline as my behaviour began to change. For example, one of my coping mechanisms was to go and have a coffee at Tim Horton's every morning. It was a nice break from a usually hectic morning routine with getting the girls off to school before I began work. I tried to time my "visits" to Tim Horton's so I could better help Pat. The next biggest challenge to our relationship was the money. Pat has always maintained our finances, usually in her head, and my unrecorded personal expenditures were throwing off her calculations. I started using a whiteboard to record my weekly cash expenses, and this helped reduce Pat's stress. I knew that I needed to change my traditional coping methods because they were no longer adequate or acceptable for a family in crisis. Change became a necessity; and hence my agreement to see the counsellor at the cancer clinic.

After the initial visits with the counsellor, I found the changes stalling. The sessions became more of an opportunity to vent my emotions than to discuss how I could become a better parent, husband and friend. Nevertheless, venting was beneficial because there really was no one else with whom I could completely share all of my pent-up emotions. So I was often alone with my feelings of inadequacy and frustration. I also believe that by relieving some of this emotional pressure, it enabled me to see the way forward a bit more clearly.

I continued the counselling sessions for a few months but stopped going after the end of Pat's chemo. After all, the worst was now over...right? Wrong! While we all thought the surgery and radiation would be easier, they were actually the hardest part of the treatment. *By February 24, 2009, I had completed 24,552 stitches.*

On March 6, 2009, I took Pat to St. Joe's for her surgery. After the surgery was completed, Dr. Holiday announced to me that Pat was okay. The surgery went well. He "got it all." Dr. Holiday put in two drains (one for each side) and set up home-care visits over the next couple of weeks. Since Pat had day surgery, we left for home about 4:00 p.m. We thought it would be fine. Pat felt a bit of discomfort but no pain. We felt relieved!

Jodi, a very close friend of Pat's whom she had known since her undergraduate university days, came from Peterborough to stay with her overnight. I slept in another room that night and did not realize that Pat had a hematoma (a bleed). Fortunately Eliza and Leonie were spending the night at the home of Pat's nephew and niece (Mike and Michelle). Jodi took Pat to the emergency room the next day. I took the girls to a hotel overnight directly from Mike and Michelle's home and called to see how Pat was later that evening. By the time I returned home the next day, everything seemed fine.

On the Monday, March 9, 2009, I sent the following email to a friend:

141

Pat's surgery went very well. She was in surgery for just over two hours, followed by two hours in recovery and then two hours in the surgical "day care." We left the hospital around 4:00 p.m. on Friday. She didn't feel any pain probably because the surgeon putting in a pain block or killing the nerve. Jodi, a long-time friend who is also a nurse, came from Peterborough to spend the weekend and she was a wonderful help. There was some post-surgery bleeding that concerned Pat enough for her to go to emergency Saturday evening. Jodi took her because I needed to pick up Eliza and Leonie from Pat's nephew's house and take them to the hotel where we stayed Saturday night. The doctor wasn't concerned about it, stating that there appeared to be some post-surgery bleeding probably caused by excessive movement (which in reality couldn't be avoided). The surgeon called Sunday morning having heard about the "bruising" and felt that Pat's platelets, while good, were probably not working as well as they should due to the chemo.

I arrived home with the girls around noon on Sunday, and they were very glad to see their mom looking so well (and she looked so much better than on Saturday). She was sitting downstairs in the sunroom and was feeling hungry enough to eat. Jodi left Sunday afternoon and Lesley, another friend who lives in London, came over to help and spent the afternoon and evening. I picked up Karen, a friend who lives in Toronto, from the train station at 6:45 p.m., and she is staying with us until Thursday morning. So, as you can see, there hasn't been a shortage of help.

Homecare was arranged, but it became an issue as there was no apparent set time for them to visit. Pat felt like a prisoner, never knowing when they would appear to change her dressings. As a nurse, Pat was also skeptical that they were following proper protocols regarding the cleaning of the wound site and the drain. Within a week, there was a problem with the drain on Pat's right side with a buildup of what appeared to be "pus" inside the tube. There was also increased pain around the site, and the skin became very pink. On March 15th, Pat was feeling chilled. Afraid of sepsis, she asked me to take her to Emergency. Luckily it was Sunday afternoon, and Lesley came to be with the girls. After waiting for a few hours, Pat was checked and the doctors decided to keep her overnight.

Pat was discharged from the hospital the next morning, and we hoped that this was now behind us. So much for that hope! On Monday evening, Pat had the "chills" again and we returned to Emergency. We had to wait a few hours before being seen by a doctor. There was a different team on this evening, and they appeared to be quite indifferent, chatting around the desk. The resident surgeon on call checked on Pat and basically dismissed her concerns as minor. After consultation with Dr. Holiday, they did decide to again keep her overnight. Even though Pat was crying when I left around 10:30 p.m., I had to return home to Eliza and Leonie. I called the hospital on Tuesday and found that Pat did have sepsis (bacteria in the blood) and that she needed to stay in the hospital for a few days. The few days turned into a week. March break from school was very stressful for the girls because Pat was in hospital. I took the week off work to be with them. It is very difficult when you don't have people who can actually come and stay to help when there is a crisis. It was a very long week!

With the crisis of sepsis behind us, we moved to the new challenge of radiation, which started on April 6th. Since radiation treatment was five days a week for six weeks, Pat, her usual organized self, had arranged for drivers to take her to the cancer clinic back in January and February. I would drive once a week to be with Pat during her weekly meeting with Dr. Pereira, her radiology oncologist. I was also the back up when someone couldn't make it on a particular day.

Initially the radiation treatments went well, with very little visible affect. However, within two weeks, Pat's skin was turning red and after a month it was starting to blister. She was applying special burn cream that helped a great deal, but her skin was breaking down more and more quickly with each treatment. After twenty-five treatments, she couldn't wear any clothes against her skin and walking was difficult. The pain was constant. The radiologist offered to delay treatment, but Pat said no – she wanted it finished to minimize the chance of the cancer recurring. Her flesh looked like raw hamburger! The radiation had been so intense that it went completely through her and burned her back! *By June 10, 2009 I had completed 31,680 stitches.*

On June 23, 2009, I sent the following email to my Aunt in England:

Hi Audrey:

I apologize for not communicating more often over the past few months, but I have simply not had the time or the energy while dealing with everything else going on at work but especially at home. I have a few minutes before I head home from work, so I thought that I would send a quick email to update you on how we are doing after the intensive nine months we have just gone through with Pat's breast cancer and all of the treatments. She completed the daily radiation treatments at the end of May and by the end of the thirty sessions her chest looked like raw hamburger. The radiation burn actually went right through her and was visible on her back. She had to use Epsom salts every day to clean the wound and then use this special cream that is used to treat severe burn patients.

Since the end of treatment time, the family is recovering, although a lot slower than we would prefer. In many ways, the few weeks after her treatment ended were some of the worst days that she had. She was getting depressed and irritable, primarily due to a couple of the drugs that she needed during treatments but could stop once treatment ended. One of the withdrawal side effects were depression and irritability. Also, shifting from "treatment" to "recovery" required a shift in thinking, both for her and the family.

She also suffered from sciatica due to her posture during radiation treatment (she had to hunch over to keep her clothing away from the burn) and from how she was positioned on the radiation table. She was unable to walk or bend over for three weeks. While that is getting better, she is still feeling exhausted, although she does have fleeting moments of energy when she is able to work and do things around the house. Did you feel completely exhausted after your cancer treatments? How long did it take you to feel that you had the energy to start doing things again, such as gardening? Our oncologist estimates that it could take twelve to fourteen months before Pat is back to feeling 100 percent (or as close as she will get)

I attended a conference in Winnipeg at the end of May and another the following week, mistakenly believing that because Pat's treatments were over, she would start feeling better right away—wrong!! She was exhausted both mentally and physically, and she found the time that I was gone very challenging, especially due to the sciatica and exhaustion. Fortunately, Leonie is doing much better after struggling mightily with Pat's cancer. Eliza is having challenges right now because we believe she sublimated her feelings about cancer by transferring them to school. Over the past few weeks she has become more remote and non-communicative. But she is now starting to let her emotions out and her feelings about the cancer without really knowing how to express them to us. At the same time, she is entering a new phase of her life as she graduates from grade eight and looks forward to starting high school in the fall. Fortunately she has an excellent relationship with Pat, which will help her get through this troubling time in her life.

While the last couple of weeks have definitely seen an improvement in Pat's overall health, she is feeling frustrated that she can't do more. She has periods where there is enough energy to work and get things done around the house but they are fleeting and often leave her exhausted. This hasn't stopped her from organizing more renovations for the house. As you may recall, we had a large (15' x

20') sunroom built last year that dramatically changed the main floor of our house. Her nephew, Mike, is currently replacing our soffits and facia. This will be followed up with a contractor installing new eavestroughs. Then he will be fixing the wiring in the three bedrooms, which will be followed up by yet another contractor blowing in enough insulation to raise the R value to 50.

It took over a month for Pat to start feeling well enough to begin walking again. I would walk her around our crescent. The recovery, while slow, was steady. As she started feeling better, her attention turned back to the family and our continuing inability to get along as well as we should. Eliza and I were back to squabbling, usually over her procrastination in picking up after herself. Leonie, while less needy, still needed her mom nearly every evening. I was drifting back to "my cave" in the basement and my cross stitch. Pat said she was beginning to hate the cross stitch picture she had selected because it was taking me away from the family. It was time for family counselling.

We were a family in crisis! Tremendous progress had been made over the past several months but it was primarily between Pat and me and between the girls and me. There were still issues between Pat and the girls, who expected everything to go back to normal now that her treatment was over. Again there was competition for Pat's limited time and energy that exhausted her even more. The girls were "sniping" at each other even more now, and the arguments between Eliza and me began escalating again, although I was taking a more adult role. I had again begun retreating to my "cave," the basement, in the evenings. Pat was exhausted! I was exhausted! The girls were angry, and school was ending!

The family counselling sessions were extremely valuable, especially for Pat and Eliza. The counsellor, Pirie, basically told Pat to "stop picking up the papers," which meant that she should not assume the responsibility for everything that happens in the household. Due to Pat's childhood and the lack of safety and security, she was over vigilant and would either do things herself or "nag" us to get household tasks done. Conversely, the counsellor recommended that I "get out of my cave" and take a more active role in the household. Sometimes when you hear things from someone outside the family with whom you are able to relate, it actually resonates and positive changes can occur. Since the counsellor had a family and was male, Pat thought that I saw him as a "positive father image," providing sage advice that was not available elsewhere. This was especially helpful with helping me develop a closer relationship with my teenage daughter. Listening to how he had interacted with his teenage children, provided me with a greater understanding of how to interact with Eliza.

While the counsellor focused on Pat to help her relax more within the family, he also focused on Eliza to get her to communicate more during the counselling session. He wanted her to explain how she felt and how she could help the family. Interestingly, Leonie was mostly quiet during the counselling sessions, and the counsellor, didn't see a need to get her to talk too much. I think he recognized, as did the rest of us, that Leonie was healing much faster than the rest of us.

The question that most concerned Pat was would the family revert back to its "old ways" once the counselling sessions ended or would they be the springboard to a closer and more respectful relationship. The first test would be vacation at the cottage. "The cottage" is located on Mississippi Lake near Carleton Place and is owned by Bruce and Bev. Bruce is a fellow Rotarian and was serving on the board of directors during this time. He and Bev offered the cottage to us each summer for a couple of weeks, at no cost. It was secluded, quiet and had limited amenities (no cable or satellite) to entertain electronically savvy children.

For the first time in the five years that we had vacationed at the cottage, I didn't spend a lot of time thinking about work. In previous years, I would use the proximity to Ottawa as an opportunity to meet some government officials or attend Rotary functions. This time I only made one excursion into Ottawa with Bruce to meet with the Afghanistan Pakistan Task Force staff and joined Bruce at his weekly Rotary meeting. The rest of the time I devoted to spending with the family. Pat and I would walk in the morning (four km). I learned from bitter experience that I am allergic to deer fly bites, so, I prepared for these walks by covering myself head to toe and brandishing an electric fly swatter. I figured that I would rather sweat than get bitten.

In the afternoon, I would spend time with the girls in the lake or paddling in the blow-up dinghy. Pat and I would prepare the meals, and I would often wash the dishes. There is something very therapeutic about washing dishes by hand, something that is lost with the dishwasher. Evenings were spent reading, doing cross-stitch or just relaxing on the deck.

Since I have always had trouble sleeping at the cottage, I would move myself to the couch on the main floor. This also meant that I woke up very early, often at first light. In previous years, I would travel the thirteen km to the Tim Horton's in Carleton Place for a coffee and bagel. This year we made a wonderful discovery in the small village of Almonte, about twenty km from the cottage—Baker Bob's! It was a small local bakery that served coffee that was just as good as "Timmy's" and had fresh baked croissants. It replaced Tim Horton's and became my early morning destination every morning of our stay. I even got to know the staff and "Baker Bob" himself. Pat had found Baker Bob's while we were exploring the villages close to the cottage the day after we arrived. In previous years, we would go to Smith Falls and visit the Hershey's factory or visit Perth, but Hershey's had closed and Perth was losing its charm. We were looking for other places to visit. We also discovered that Almonte hosted "Puppets Up," a weekend festival that invited puppeteers from around the world to stage puppet shows. It was scheduled for the next weekend, and while Pat and Eliza weren't overly interested, Leonie was very excited about attending this event. She and I went Saturday morning, expecting to only be there for a couple of hours. We ended up staying most of the day because she was enjoying it so much and, truth be told, so was I.

Eliza had just completed her bronze cross in the summer, which is one step away from becoming certified as a lifeguard. Completing this course at the age of thirteen was a tremendous feat as usually only teenagers between fourteen and sixteen take this course. At the cottage, Eliza didn't think she needed to wear a life jacket while swimming. Pat and I reluctantly agreed (our little girl was growing up) but with limitations. She couldn't swim too far from the shore unless one of us was with her. She wanted to swim around the island, which was about 100 meters from the shore, and we agreed but only if I was with her in the paddle boat or inflatable dinghy. We set out, her swimming and me paddling the inflatable dinghy. She was much better at swimming than I was at paddling. She had no trouble circumventing the island and sometimes had to wait for me to catch up to her.

Both girls wanted me to join them in the water, and so during one of the warm sunny days, reluctantly I agreed. We had purchased an inflatable water trampoline, and the girls had a lot of fun jumping and diving from it. They also wanted me to jump on the trampoline. From the shore it looked easy, but once I swam out to it, I realized I had to pull myself out of the water without tipping over the trampoline. The only way I could do it was to pull myself out of the water and over the trampoline like a whale at Marineland. Once I had most of my weight on the trampoline, I could squirm to the point where I could stand up. I also discovered that floating trampolines are not very stable, especially for someone over 200 pounds. Needless to say, I did several "headers" into the lake. This was captured on video that the girls would watch or share with friends and guests when they wanted a good laugh.

Pat was still very tired, but for the first time she felt that I was with the family both physically and emotionally. The skirmishes with Eliza were fewer and farther between, and I believe that we had started to bond more closely together as a family.

Change can come suddenly—like an epiphany—or sometimes so slowly you aren't aware that a change is taking place. My change towards my family was very slow. In fact I was not really aware that a change was taking place, but Pat saw it, and from time to time she would comment on how much better we were getting along as a family. Thank you, Pirie. *By August 21, 2009 I had completed 35,640 stitches.*

Even though I was making progress, I believe that my path to becoming more connected to my family was often obscured and obstructed by the pressures and stress of work. At work, our funding approval was further delayed with the government requests for more information or changes to the proposal. I understood that compliance would make us a much more effective organization. The organization received a "non-funded" extension of its current agreement with the government until November 30, 2009, leading to feelings of financial stress at work. All of the delays in funding, however, made me begin to question if I would soon need to seek other employment. At the same time, Pat was informed that the funding for her program would cease in May 2010. The situation was even more difficult because Pat was suffering from a clinical depression. At first we all thought this was caused by the notification that she would be losing "the best job in the world" in May and by her fears around who would hire a cancer "victim." Needless to say, it was a very stressful Christmas. *By January 2, 2010 I had completed 42,768 stitches.*

I have always said to Pat that for me, the New Year doesn't start until February 1st. My "logic" in this thinking is that January is the time when we have to pay the bills for the gifts and "good times" we enjoy in December with Christmas and New Year's festivities. Knowing that you have to pay for the previous month's fun seems like a very poor way to start a new year. Pat has often laughed at my changing of the calendar, but starting 2010 on February 1st was a very good idea. January was still very stressful between Pat's continuing depression and my work-related stress. Eliza's anxiety about school and exams was escalating, and Leonie was again having difficulties at school with friends.

By the beginning of February, things were turning around for us as a family. Pat went on a mild anti-depressant and almost immediately began feeling better. Eliza "aced" her exams, and Leonie found a new "best" friend. As for me, the government granted us another funded extension with more money and reiterated how much they wanted to keep us as a partner. I went on a mild anti-depressant to help me feel better for a couple of weeks, and it worked.

Eliza's high school is on the semester system, so after exams were finished, she would start four new courses. One of these was geography. Both Pat and Eliza are "geographically challenged," so this would be the first opportunity for me to help Eliza with her homework and to further build our bond that had gradually been improving since the summer. The first "test" came in March with one of the first major quizzes. Eliza had missed a week of school due to a severe cold and had missed the test, but was given the opportunity to write it when she came back. I helped her study and introduced some extrapolated questions from the material. At the time she said that they wouldn't be on the quiz and only answered my questions reluctantly. However, two of my questions were on the test and, because we had studied them, she was able to answer them correctly! I think, for the first time, Eliza realized that I had some gifts that could help her with school. Since then, Eliza has told Pat a few times that she would rather have Dad help her to to study geography and to do research. *By March 13, 2010, I had completed 49,104 stitches, representing a completion of one-third of the picture, leaving only 98,208 stitches left to go!*

By March 2010, Eliza and I were still having skirmishes and I was still struggling to find the balance between loving her and being frustrated by what she had done or left undone. However, overall we are learning to not only love each other but to also like each other. Pat noticed this and commented on how much I had changed. Interestingly, I don't feel like I am changing, which must mean that the change is taking place subconsciously, almost at a "subatomic" level. I do notice that I enjoy being around the family a lot more than I used to and am less obsessive with work and my cross-stitch. I am feeling more comfortable with myself, understanding that "to err is human" and we are all jerks sometimes.

Reflections:

The peaceable kingdom, noted in Isaiah, is a metaphor for heaven without hate, conflict or the need to "feed off of one another." While it represents a utopia that is not realistic for our world, it provides a guide for how we should lead our lives. Conflict is part of the human condition. History teaches us that violence seldom leads to a permanent solution. Each new generation seems to have to learn history's lessons again and again. Human conflict is inflicted externally, upon each other, but also internally as we struggle to find our place in this world.

As a student of history, I am very aware of the many conflicts throughout the ages. However, it is only by experiencing Pat's journey through "the shadow of death" that I faced my inner conflicts. I am more aware that I need to be accepted by the greater community, which led to my involvement in several community organizations, ranging from committee chair to a volunteer. It was very challenging to give up these activities to devote more time to my family. Between September 2008 and December 2008, I was able to divest myself of most of my community activities, but I found that I was suffering from feelings of guilt because I was letting others down. Guilt? Why would I feel this way? I had difficulties setting priorities when it was obvious that my family should come first, especially during this time of crisis.

The path to enlightenment is often tortuous, twisted and tangled, and my struggle to understand why I felt guilt was no different. I came to the realization through this inner conflict that I did have a much higher need for approval from the outside community than from my own family. Upon reflection and many lengthy discussions with Pat, I came to the understanding that these feelings were unresolved issues from my adolescence. I never felt appreciated within my nuclear family. Whether or not that is true is immaterial; it was what I "felt." In order to gain acceptance and be appreciated, I turned to people outside the family. In many ways, I became a "chameleon," adapting my personality to meet the perceived expectations of those around me. Needless to say, this was not a very successful strategy. I learned to disengage my emotions because I believed that being emotional around my family was an invitation to be hurt. With people outside of the family, the danger was limited because I could choose what to share and if the relationship became too personal or emotional, it was easy to "walk away."

With Pat's support, I made tremendous progress in understanding the role my childhood played in determining the path I took during my adulthood. However, I was still a "work in progress," and the family health crisis forcibly propelled me into working on the two most critical areas where I needed to grow: placing the family first and becoming more closely attached to my emotions at an adult level.

The more I divested myself of community distractions, the easier it became to put the family first. However, I was never fully successful due to the increasing stress and workload of my job. While Pat understood, most of the time, my work was a contentious issue between us. The girls seldom understood that I had to be at work or had to travel for work, especially since their mom was working from home. My absences from home were acutely felt by the rest of the family and increased my level of guilt and stress. However, there were times when I travelled for work that I was able to "suspend reality" and focus on the business at hand. This was very empowering as I felt completely disempowered at home. I couldn't heal Pat! I tried to understand the turmoil, confusion, and anger from the girls, but I was still not attached to my emotions. I was unable to comfort! In fact I didn't even know how to even start to offer comfort. I did "tactile" things such as get the groceries, cook and clean up whenever possible, run errands, take Pat to her appointments. I comforted myself by "counting" my progress on my cross stitch.

Emotions! There is no escape from them. No matter how much you deny them or subjugate them to logic, they will find you. I didn't find my emotions—Eliza found them for me and it wasn't pretty! Well-adjusted teenagers seldom suffer from the inability to voice their feelings or state their opinions. True, they often come from the perspective of self-interest, but that is part of the transition from childhood to adulthood. Teenagers are developing an understanding of their place in the world. This often brings grief and frustration to well-intentioned parents who both understand the need for their teenager to take these development steps but are often the target of their teenager's anger and frustrations towards the world.

This grief and frustration is amplified when the teenager has been well taught in the art of debating by her mother. This is further exacerbated when she is brighter than her father with a quickness of tongue that leaves him reeling, stammering for some kind of appropriate response and failing miserably. As I recently mentioned to friends, arguing with Eliza is like going to a gun battle armed only with a putty knife.

While I am sure that this situation is fairly common between adolescents and their parents, what is interesting for our story is how I responded to always losing these arguments. I regressed to a teenager myself! Pat often felt that she had two adolescents in the house. The progression of one of our arguments was like a three-act play. The first act was the disagreement and the bantering back and forth (usually around two to three minutes). There was no resolution during this act, only the clarification of the demarcation line. The second act was the entrenchment of our respective positions, from which we would hurl recriminations at each other in steadily escalating voices (usually for around five minutes). The third act ended in one of two ways. I would get so angry and upset that I would stomp out of the house and go for a lengthy walk, muttering the entire time. The other way was for Pat to intervene and tell us to stop squabbling like a couple of children. Eliza and I would both accuse Pat of taking the other person's side. Both endings often resulted in a reconciliation meeting between Eliza and me mediated by Pat.

Because Pat felt that her family was killing her faster than the cancer, I made the decision to build a stronger bond with Eliza as a parent. This wasn't easy, and I needed outside help from professional counsellors to come to the realization that if I wanted a relationship with Eliza, I needed to be the instigator. Pat has often stated that we, as parents, have a limited shelf life before our influence is replaced by friends. Eliza will be moving on to university within three years and creating her own life separate from that of her parents. The clock is ticking, and time is running out for me to have a healthy, interactive relationship with her.

The most valuable lessons that I have learned over the past two years when dealing with family are:
* Family priorities surpass all other priorities. After all, family is forever, while everything else is transitory. Guilt is a tool, often employed to avoid personal development. Personal development requires that we reflect upon who we are and move to make changes that will give us greater understanding of ourselves. Many people find this frightening and will attempt to maintain their comfortable yet often dysfunctional personal paradigm at all costs.
* You need to accept that you will never "win" an argument or power struggle with a teenager. Hopefully you have enough influence to provide a positive guiding hand for their further development.

* Pick your battles. Most arguments are over petty, small issues that are often quickly forgotten. The key is to not let the small issues escalate into an all out war. The parent never wins because the teenager is not bound by the same social rules. Try not to react to the sharpness of voice, the inappropriate language or the dramatic mood swings. They are part of this stage called adolescence that will pass (or so I am told). It is important to hear your teenager and understand her world, which is something I am still struggling to do on a consistent basis.

* Trust your emotions to your family. Love means you will feel cared for and cherished.

The Peaceable Kingdom:

It is only after the crisis has passed that you can sit back and reflect upon what has happened and contemplate whether it has changed your worldview. The peaceable kingdom verse in Isaiah 11:6 initially resonated with me because this was the cross stitch picture I was creating. Some of the mental images that can be drawn from this verse and from the picture are of the cancer, represented by the lion and the leopard, being tamed by the family, represented by the "kid." Being led by a "little child" brings to mind the birth of Jesus as the incarnation of something new and better for the world. We, as a family, are forever changed from having experienced this brush with death. I believe we will have more compassion and caring for others and ourselves. The imagery also represents my need for inner peace as I suffered through the inner turmoil, conflicts, stresses and worries brought about by Pat's breast cancer.

"The wolf shall also dwell with the lamb and the leopard shall lie down with the kid" represents cancer as the

wolf and leopard and our family as the lamb and kid. Sometimes cancer is not diagnosed until after it has metastasized (spread) to several places in the body and is attacking you like a pack of ravenous wolves. Other times it can sneak up on you like a leopard and attack silently with no warning in only one part of your body. In either case, the attack can be deadly if not discovered in time. Our cancer was like the leopard, silently attacking Pat while disguising itself as mastitis until it was almost too late. My peaceable kingdom would only come with accepting that the cancer has been fought and defeated and will probably never return. Cancer was the focus of our lives during this journey. We learned to realize that it touches virtually everyone at some time and that most people survive and continue to live long and productive lives.

Cancer brings out the best and worst in people. Some friends and family were afraid for us but couldn't help. Others, who were just as afraid, were able to be there whenever they were needed. Pat had a small cadre of friends whom she could rely upon to help her, and by helping Pat, they were helping me and the girls. Karen, Lesley, Kate, Jodi and Elaine deserve special mention for the support they provided on a daily, weekly or monthly basis. There is a saying that every dark cloud has a silver lining. The clouds that encompassed our family during 2008 and 2009 have never looked so dark or menacing. The silver lining is the friends that helped and the understanding each of us gained about each other. Because of this life-threatening experience, we have a much closer bond as a family than ever before. As a person, I am more complete! I still have insecurities, and I will do things that will label me as "a jerk," but overall I am more at peace with myself and with my life as a husband

and father. Progress towards the "Peaceable Kingdom" is a pretty good outcome, during two of the most difficult years of my life.

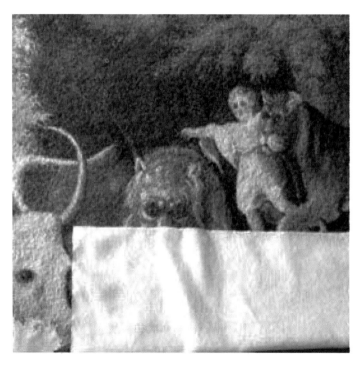

Peaceable Kingdom unfolding—54,000 stiches completed, only 96,000 to go

Chapter 8

Leonie's Chapter Two
Age 10

It has been one year since my mom got cancer. It still feels hard when I watch my mom sitting on the couch and feeling sad. It makes me very nervous. I don't like to talk about it at all.

Now I'm going to school. I don't have to go to the school counsellor as much now I'm more relaxed. I do feel like I want to cry when someone brings it up.

During all of last year we went to a family counsellor. Our counsellor's name was Pirie. Me and Eliza did not say much at all. Mom and Dad said a lot. Eliza did not like to go to the counsellor. Then Mom brought up the fights. Dad and Eliza had a lot. Eliza had a lot to say about that and so did Dad. Eliza did not have to say a lot about Mom or me until Mom said something. Pirie finally got Eliza to say what she wanted to say. The day we were done with family counselling, Eliza was happy to go. I really liked Pirie after we were done. I think there was a difference in our family.

A couple months later my gerbil, Lela, died. I was really sad for a couple days, then my mom said to go to the pet store and figure out what animal lives long. We ended up getting a hamster. I named him Popcorn. Actually my sister came up with the name. I love him. I have had him for one year, and I can actually hold him without him running away. Sometimes when he is tired, I quietly pick him up and put him on my lap. I put a blanket over my lap. When I look at my lap in five minutes or so, he's there and he is still sleeping.

Chapter 9

Easter Saturday: In the Tomb Recovery

The disciples were hidden away feeling afraid on Easter Saturday. They were mourning the loss of a loved one and leader and feeling helpless. I also felt emotionally and physically broken and helpless, wanting desperately to hide from the world. When is it really safe to come out?

On Easter Saturday, there needs to be a time for lamentations. Maybe you have to go through the tomb to heal; maybe the tears of lamentation water the body to help it heal. The time in the tomb or hidden in the upper room feels like forever. Will the losses and tears ever end?

June, 2009

I always thought that chemo would be the hardest step of the journey with cancer. That idea seems so naive and remote now. After five months of complications, I could not get beyond the fear that "another shoe would drop" and my life would again be in peril. Life felt pressured, and I continued to push myself, even though in hindsight I wish that I hadn't.

In June, my first step towards healing was to begin meditation sessions at Wellspring in London (a support centre for people with cancer and their families). In the past, I had never been successful at practicing mediation; nevertheless, I believed that if I didn't change the way I was living, I was sure the cancer would return.

In the meditation group, we all silently say metta. Metta comes out of the Buddhist philosophy of sowing the seeds of intention for loving kindness. Over 2,500 years ago, the Buddha gave his disciples the ritual of metta as an antidote for fear. During metta you repeat the following phrases:

> May I be safe from inner and outer harm;
> May I be happy just the way I am;
> May I be healthy, may my body serve me well; and
> May I be peaceful and at ease.

First I said metta for myself because the Buddha says there is no one more deserving of loving kindness than you. Nevertheless, I had a great deal of trouble saying metta for myself. I would say the words, but they felt empty. The nice part about metta, though, is you are just sowing the seeds of intention and you don't have to believe that it is happening now. You don't even have to believe it *should* happen; just believe that it *may* happen in the future.

We begin the meditation with the "forgiveness." We ask forgiveness of others whom we may have hurt; we forgive those who may have hurt us; and we forgive ourselves. I found it much easier to find it in my heart to quietly ask for forgiveness from others and to forgive others than to forgive myself. Over time, I would think about all the mistakes I had made that may have caused harm to others. I would visualize asking them for forgiveness and wait for a response. Sometimes I had to visualize myself apologizing many times until I felt that the person had forgiven me (if only in my mind). The second part of forgiving others was fairly easy since I had been letting go of past "slights" or "harms" since I had been diagnosed with cancer. I knew that I could ill afford to expend my energy on anger and resentments when it was needed for healing. A major positive change was that I was able to say metta for someone with whom I harboured difficult feelings within moments of being upset. I discovered it was difficult to say metta and be angry at the same time. It has become a big part of my life and helps me feel calmer.

The area in which I had the most difficulty was trying to forgive myself. I still had a long list of things for which I thought I needed to forgive myself. For example, I need forgiveness for being so anxious my whole life, secondly for carrying resentment my whole life about being neglected as a child, and thirdly, for wanting recognition, often for my work. When I was successful, forgiving myself brought a sense of peace rather than just energy management (not feeling like you are wasting energy). I am still working on forgiving myself.

I wondered why it was so easy for me to say metta for other people and so difficult to say it for myself. In the beginning, I pretended I was in the group looking down at myself. I was trying to learn to treat myself as I have treated others. I never really acknowledged it may have been an issue of self-worth. I now look back and realize that children often learn to value themselves through the love of their parents. Being orphaned at age five, I probably never really reached the stage of self-acceptance since I rarely heard affirming messages saying I was worthwhile.

Throughout my career, I have taught people how to reach their potential. Now I need to take my own advice!

As time progressed, I integrated my Christian beliefs into the metta. After we said the forgiveness and began metta, I would recite the Lord's Prayer. I focused on the lines "Forgive us our trespasses as we forgive the trespasses of others." I also said "the Lord is my Shepherd" because this psalm always seems to calm my emotions. These prayers helped me "focus" at the beginning of meditation.

The second part of meditation is guided imagery. I always hated these exercises in nursing school, but I now tried to visualize my body and soul healing. The guided imagery was about twenty minutes long, but most of the time I would tune out our leader (Deborah) with her blessing and go on the path of healing that I heard and saw in my own mind. I would often go back to very lonely and sad times in my childhood and comfort my inner child while imagining me mothering myself as a child. I used the same techniques that I use with Eliza and Leonie, listening to my childhood woes and then comforting myself. Miraculously, many of these very sad memories of neglect started to fade in their capacity to hurt me. Over time I became better and better at achieving a meditative state, so mediation became my two most important hours of the week. It was clear I was healing both physically and emotionally.

Throughout my treatment, I managed to work and use sick time to continue working, thanks to a very understanding employer. Working helped me feel productive and avoid the crippling thoughts and fears of dying. After my radiation treatments were over, I began to really notice how exhausted I was and acknowledged that I had pushed myself beyond reason, for example, working while bedridden in tremendous pain from the radiation burn. Nevertheless in June, I went into the health unit to attend some meetings, even though I could hardly walk and sit. These meetings were both physically and emotionally painful. Unfortunately, people noticed and brought some omissions in my work to my attention and I started to cry. Given all of the complications in my illness, I finally admitted to myself that my best just wasn't good enough.

I continued to be reflective about what I needed to do to facilitate my recovery. My biggest revelation was that I needed Kevin, Eliza and Leonie to recover first! I realized I would never be able to recover before them because they needed so much of my energy. Over the past ten months, I had built up so much anger inside because they were not able to rise above their own needs while I clearly was very ill. I finally accepted that there is no answer to the kind of anger and frustration that I felt towards my family. The most healing thing to do was to forgive and then try again because while they fell short, I knew everyone had tried their best to help.

Physically, I knew that I needed more sleep. A few months earlier, Kevin kindly volunteered to sleep in a bed in the basement because his snoring literally "shook the walls" and I just couldn't sleep with the noise. Instead of sleeping alone, however, Leonie became my bedfellow. Leonie often slept with me during my treatment because she was so distressed and needed reassurance that I was still alive and with her. I am sure that some people would be shocked if they knew that Leonie was sleeping with me. Nevertheless, if Leonie didn't sleep, she became more fretful and irritable the next day and I would have more difficulty coping. Leonie slept with me because we did what we needed to do, in the moment, to get through. After treatment was over, however, I realized I would enjoy more rest if she was sleeping in her own bed. Now with Leonie at age ten, we were using the Ferber method of letting the child cry herself to sleep with timed comforting. My heart felt like it was breaking when I heard her sob as she was going to sleep. Thus when Leonie asked for a gerbil to be her friend when she was sad, Kevin and I readily agreed to buying each of the girls a gerbil (Lela and Corona). The little rodents helped the girls adjust and feel better.

By July, I really started to see some healing in Leonie. She began to laugh and sing around the house again; she was much more animated, and she was very glad to physically see I was getting better. Leonie wore her anger, sadness and grief on her sleeve the whole period and, in hindsight, I think that Leonie, at ten years of age, was the wisest of us all. She was honest about her feelings and didn't hide them. She wrote her story "A Scary Thought" in May, 2009. She understood that it would still be a while before I recovered, but she didn't fear my imminent death all the time now. I could tell she was gaining some perspective on healing way beyond her years.

In June, I was surprised to see Eliza becoming more irritable and angry. She also began having complaints of nausea and stomach aches. When I asked how she was feeling, she eventually told me she had "buried" her pent up emotions when I was so sick because she did not want to add to my burden. In hindsight, Eliza found it easier to worry about the small stuff, like "Am I academic material?" rather than the bigger question "Will my mother die?" I told her that all of my friends were experiencing these feelings as well. Everyone was trying to be optimistic, but they were still very frightened inside. We began addressing her anger and distress, but we were a far cry from completely resolving these distressing symptoms.

In June, Eliza graduated from grade eight. I had always thought I would get Eliza pearls for her grade twelve graduation, but since I was very afraid that I would not live until her grade twelve graduation, I decided I needed to do it now. Because I had fond memories of living spontaneously in my twenties and thirties, I decided to try to learn again how to live in the moment, beginning with the pearls. Thus, I asked Eliza's godmothers if they would like to go shopping to get Eliza pearls. First we went out to dinner and then we agreed to go to only one store so I did not over tire myself. Eliza enjoyed trying on numerous pieces of jewellery before she chose her pearl necklace, and her godmothers bought her matching earrings. I was very tired by the time we got home, but I was pleased I was able to give Eliza this special evening.

Later that month, I went to Eliza's graduation. I wanted to make it a great night for Eliza, even though I felt very tired and had to overcome my self-consciousness about my appearance (I had very straggly hair, no eyebrows, very few eyelashes and very large dark circles under my eyes). First, Eliza and I went to our hairdresser Farzaneh in the afternoon to have her hair done. Eliza looked splendid. We had a celebratory dinner prior to the ceremony with my nephew, Mike and his wife Michelle (who was almost nine months pregnant) and my sister and niece.

Kevin dropped me off at the door of the high school where the ceremony was being held, so I wouldn't have far to walk. I averted my gaze when I thought people were staring at me because I was so self-conscious about my appearance; I tried to camouflage my belief that my personality was just a shadow of its former self. Some of Eliza's friends' parents asked me how I was, and I felt very uncomfortable lying to them by saying that I was okay. The ceremony was over by 8:15 p.m., and Eliza went to the dance. I went home pleased I could share her special night.

At the end of June, Kate retired as the priest of her church. She had made such a contribution as a parish priest, but she wanted more time with her family. We attended her final service. I sincerely hoped that they would find someone who could remotely compare to Kate. I knew I still needed to attend worship on Sundays to help me recover.

I really know what it was like for the disciples to miss Jesus. They must have felt lost. Who could possibly take Kate's place for me?

July 2009

Kevin and I continued to explore ways to help him better understand himself so that he wouldn't be so easily emotionally triggered by Eliza. Lesley suggested we try family therapy through the Employee Assistance Program (EAP) available through work. It was clear that Eliza was taking her anger out on her father, and Kevin responded irritably when verbally attacked. When the therapist, Pirie, asked what I wanted to achieve in therapy, I said I wanted the girls to be able to comfort themselves and I wanted everyone to help me with the domestic work so I could get some rest.

Pirie's first instructions to Kevin were to "get out of the cave" and for me "to get into the cave." I thought this was a very quaint way to tell Kevin to be more active in the family and to tell me to step back and let Kevin go into action. Kevin and Eliza began very slowly to work on their relationship, and the family counselling really helped them to resolve some of their differences.

During one session of family counselling, I wanted to bring up cancer as the "unspoken elephant" in the room. To my surprise, Kevin and the girls weren't really thinking about it. In their eyes, my treatment was over and they were moving on. I discovered that Easter Saturday was plainly over for them, and even though they weren't at the resurrection stage yet, they were busy with their current day-to-day lives. I was the one who was still stuck in Easter Saturday.

In order to get some dedicated time to myself, I decided to go to a twenty-four-hour silent retreat at Medaille House (run by Catholic nuns). On the day that I was supposed to go, I had to drag myself there because I was feeling so overwhelmed and tired. As soon as I got there, I slept, and then I read. I walked the labyrinth (a sacred walk) to see if I experienced any insights into healing. At the silent retreat, I made the decisions to begin writing my book and to learn to love and take care of myself. I brought a small granite stone home from the labyrinth to remind me of my goals. I carried this stone in my pocket as I walked around our neighbourhood. Sister C., who is the spiritual counsellor at Medaille House, said that it was a miracle that I made it through the treatment. These words helped give me a new perspective on life. She suggested that God was sending people to help me (or at least that is what I understood). I went home twenty-four hours later feeling a little better.

Even though the radiation had now been over for two months, my physical tiredness was still very pronounced. I was still afraid to walk farther than around the block in case I became tired and couldn't make it home. Occasionally, I would walk with people a little farther. Eventually, I went to my family doctor because I was afraid that the tiredness meant that the cancer was back. Dr. Kumar ordered blood work. I was terrified to get the results because I assumed the results would be bad from the damage from the chemo and radiation treatments. I started thinking about dying again and about what would happen to my family. I worried for over two weeks and made an appointment to review the results with Dr. Kumar. To my surprise everything was normal except that my white blood cells were a little low. Dr. Kumar said that was to be expected. Once again, I was overwhelmed without a reason.

I continued to be very vigilant for any signs of physical healing from my chemo, probably because I am a nurse. My nails had white rings on them that were spaced apart, showing the damage and healing between the last four chemo treatments, just like the rings inside the trunk of a tree showing the age of the tree. As my nails grew, I began to see the white rings move higher on my nails and I felt powerful each time I cut off a white ring. Eventually all of the rings were gone. In addition, some of the neuropathy (numbness and tingling in my hands and feet) was decreasing, even though my feet would burn if I walked too far. The sciatica healed, and I could walk more comfortably, but my posture was still somewhat stooped. The skin had healed in my right chest area, and there were no more open wounds. The hematoma on my left chest area was absorbed into my body and the lump disappeared. Even though the incision line and my right armpit were still quite numb, I could now feel my outer arm between my right elbow and the middle aspect of my outer arm that had previously been numb. It was clear my body was healing, and I felt quite pleased with these positive changes.

I wondered if Jesus noticed each of the physical changes when he was healing in the tomb.

I continued to meditate twice a week. I still struggled to say metta for myself, but the healing reflection made me feel more confident that I could and would heal further. My two hours of meditation began to feel "sacred," the only two hours of the week when I was convinced that I was really helping myself. One person in my meditation group said that she takes two-hour baths to relax. I used to take two-hour baths before I married Kevin and had my children. I realized that I hadn't taken a relaxing bath for at least fifteen years.

August 2009

It was a mistake to schedule a follow-up appointment with Dr. Potvin and Dr. Powers. and then plan to leave the same day for vacation. Prior to the appointment, my mind was caught up in thinking that maybe I should have surgery to remove my ovaries, so I wouldn't need to be on the estrogen suppressant anymore. I ruminated about this for over a week, but when I mentioned it to both doctors, they immediately replied that this was a bad idea. I took their advice because I didn't really want to have surgery again. The appointment was otherwise uneventful. My only regret was that I did not have pleasure anticipating the vacation because I was too busy thinking about my ovaries instead.

On the way to the cottage, we stopped at Jodi's in

Peterborough, a five-hour drive away. It was so nice to see Jodi again. We had dinner, a little wine and a splendid visit. I was so tired after doctors' appointments and the trip, I had to go to bed at about 9:30 p.m. Jodi and I said goodbye the night before as she needed to leave for work early the next morning.

I was still pretty tired as we set out for the cottage the next day (a three-hour drive). Kevin and the girls were very understanding when I couldn't do anything for the first two days after arriving at the cottage. On one of our first outings, we found "Baker Bob's" in Almonte, about twenty km away from the cottage. Almost every day afterwards, Kevin drove to Baker Bob's to get his coffee and freshly baked croissant. Kevin and I had the opportunity to walk together most days (four km), which was very enjoyable. Afterwards, I would relax by the lake enjoying the peace and quiet (*He leads me beside still waters*). Eliza, who had achieved her bronze cross in July, swam in the lake beside Kevin and I who were in the paddle boat. Leonie also swam in the lake but wearing her life jacket for safety. The girls read and watched DVDs. Amazingly, this turned out to be the best vacation we ever had as a family.

Later in August, we went one more time for family counselling to bring closure to our sessions. Everyone felt that progress had been made. Eliza and Kevin were getting along better. Leonie was acting more like herself (happy, singing and fun loving). I was learning to be honest about my emotions. The family was making some progress in giving me some rest. At work, we completed a large grant report, which was another weight eased off my shoulders.

Burdens can feel like a massive big rock blocking the tomb. The big question is whether the rock that is blocking the tomb is keeping things in or keeping things out.

At the end of August, I had another bone scan, and I was pleased that I didn't get nervous until the day of the appointment. Instead of worrying about having the isotope injected this time, I was more worried about whether there would be any isotope available for the scan. The Chalk River Nuclear plant (the main source of nuclear isotopes in Canada) had closed earlier in the year. While the technician was injecting the isotope, I asked her whether the isotope came from South Africa or Holland. She thought it might have been Australian. When I came back three hours later for the actual scan, there was an equipment failure and the scan had to be rerun. I was convinced that something was terribly wrong when they ran an extra test. I thought, *How could the bone scan be normal after all that radiation?* After I worried non-stop for about two weeks, I called the cancer clinic to find out the results of the bone scan, but they couldn't share them on the phone. I called my family doctor and scheduled an appointment. The bone scan was normal; however, Dr. Pereira. told me later that month I would need to have it repeated again in six months to a year because the same spot on my sternum was still visible. I guess better safe than sorry.

September, 2009

In September, Eliza began high school and the transition went pretty smoothly. I managed to go out by myself to the "Meet the Teacher" night, when Kevin was away at a conference in Edmonton. It felt good to meet Eliza's teachers.

Eliza was actually interested in school; she was doing her homework and assignments and making some new friends.

Leonie was now in grade five and liked her teachers. She was still having trouble in math, but I was able to help her with supplementary work. She continued having sleepovers with her friends and her overall life was improving.

Even though our family showed signs of improvement, I continued to be quite fatigued and anxious. My family doctor thought that it would help if I returned to work full time so that I wouldn't worry as much. I panicked! I began reliving the trauma around the anniversary of my diagnosis, and it felt just like post-traumatic stress disorder; all of my fears of death and suffering came to the forefront. I had worked part time during my treatment, and now I despaired at the thought of working more; I knew that I just couldn't do it. The all-encompassing fatigue seemed to come out of nowhere. Therefore, I decided to go the cancer clinic to find out if I was malingering or having a normal reaction to my treatment. I wondered, *Does everyone fall apart at their anniversary date?*

I sincerely doubt that Jesus fell apart and was stressed on subsequent Good Fridays. I don't think that Jesus suffered from post-traumatic stress disorder.

M., my social worker, told me many people continue to be emotional and have physical difficulties a year or longer after treatment. Thus, I decided to begin some therapy sessions to normalize my experiences and aid in my recovery. When M. asked me what I really wanted, I said I wanted to learn to take care of myself and not push myself like I had before. I wanted to continue working three days a week until Christmas to see if I could also find some joy in my life; I wanted to find more ways to enjoy my family again; and I wanted to rest when I felt tired. M. said I was learning to listen to my body. It was good to hear this message because I have a long history of being told to slow down, but instead of resting I would say I would rest another time.

Did God and angels send messages to Jesus in the tomb? Did Jesus listen to messages in the tomb? Did Jesus only rest in the tomb?

Back in January 2009, I planned a coming-out celebration party for September 26th because I was convinced that life would be going much better by then. Dr. Potvin had said it would be a difficult year, not years. Kevin and I had organized a catered pig roast when we got married in 1990 and, it had been such a fun time, so I thought we should have another one. In January 2009, I truly thought I would be almost fully recovered by September, but I was wrong. The party was still very important because I wanted to thank people for their prayers and support. Sixty people accepted our invitation, and my goal was to talk to everyone. I had a glass of watered-down wine and greeted everyone at the door; then I talked to everyone again when they came to the buffet for food; finally, I said goodbye when people were leaving. It was just like three receiving lines at a wedding. I wanted to feel loved and loving, and that was exactly what happened. It was a glorious time. Even the rainy weather could not stop everyone from having a good time. I didn't worry about being the "hostess with the mostest" because I knew everyone would introduce themselves and get to know each other. My friend Elaine, who listened patiently to every fear during our telephone calls, came to London from Victoria just for my party. The most interesting phenomenon of the evening reminded me of Jesus at the wedding. Kevin had made wine for toasts and refreshment. We had twenty-five bottles of wine prepared. Our guests participated in the toasts, and everyone enjoyed some wine during the evening. At the end of the night, we had twenty-six bottles of wine left over. What a lovely evening!

I wonder if Jesus talked to angels in the tomb like old friends at a party. Did they reminisce about old times? Did Jesus make sure everyone had enough wine?

October 2009

Back in March, I learned that my nursing class was going to have a thirtieth year reunion in October. I decided to go and called a friend, Lois, to see if we could go together. As the date approached, I became more worried about not having the energy to go, and I didn't want to expose myself as a cancer victim. In the end, I made the decision to go for one night. Lois and I drove to Niagara-on-the-Lake, and the drive was really enjoyable. Once we arrived, I lay down for a rest in the hotel; drinks were scheduled for 6:30 p.m. I felt physically tired and self-conscious when Lois and I went to the lounge. Jodi drove me to the dinner at 7:30 p.m., but unfortunately dinner wasn't served until 9:30 p.m. By 10:00 p.m., I was feeling like I might collapse. I asked Jodi to take me back to the hotel and she did. As soon as I got into her car, I burst into tears. Jodi took me back to the hotel and I got into bed and she stayed for an hour and then I fell asleep. In the morning, I woke up feeling fine. I figured that everyone would know what had happened with me by the next morning, and they did. I had breakfast and went on a walking tour for an hour and still felt fine. Kevin came at 1:00 p.m. to take me home, but by this time I was exhausted. I did not go to the reunion to have fun; I went because I was afraid that I would not survive until the thirty-fifth reunion. I went to prove to myself that I could do it. In hindsight, I think that I should have had a glass of wine in the lounge and then gone back to my room and then to dinner. It would have limited my exposure to everyone and let me rest more. I did resolve to go to the thirty-fifth anniversary.

Massage Therapy

Since July, I had been experiencing a contracture on my right shoulder. The contracture occurred as the muscles in my chest and arm were shortening, causing my shoulder to shift unnaturally forward about five cm. As the muscles shortened in my shoulder, it became progressively more painful and I started losing the range of motion in my right arm and shoulder. It even hurt to breathe and lie on my right side. My skin felt like tissue paper from the effects of the radiation.

Luckily, Lesley introduced me to her massage therapist, Joanne. On the first visit, Joanne used an ultrasound machine to begin breaking down the scar tissue in my right chest and shoulder. I was familiar with the process of massage because I had had massage in the past that helped heal an old injury. I knew it would probably hurt while the damaged tissue was massaged, but the ultrasound machine made the process painless. It did hurt, though, when Joanne physically massaged the area.

The second visit occurred a week later. Once again, Joanne massaged the area and used the ultrasound machine.

181

At one point, Joanne pulled my right arm and I heard a click, and she said my arm bone was now in its socket. The contracture had actually shortened the chest muscles so much that it had dislocated my arm bone. I had no idea this could happen. On the fourth visit, Joanne pressed on my back during the massage and I heard another "click." This time she had put my rib back into alignment. Once again, I never realized my rib was out of place. No wonder I was in so much pain. I also began to notice that my skin was starting to heal, and I was getting more feeling back in my right armpit, right suture line, and in the back of my right arm. Joanne explained that the scar tissue was so tight it was interfering with the circulation of blood to my muscles, nerves and skin, and the breaking up of this scar tissue allowed more blood flow to the damaged tissue to facilitate healing. My skin also began to regain its natural moisture and thicken, losing its papery appearance.

On the fifth visit, my sternum (breast bone) started to return to its natural position rather than protruding like the chest of a pigeon. Some of the pain was receding and I could now have treatment every second week. On the sixth visit, Joanne was able to improve the range of motion in my right arm using a technique whereby she twisted my arm. This technique reminded me of the neighbourhood bully when I was a child when he used to twist my arm behind my back to make me cry. They both painfully twisted my arm but with completely different motives. Over the summer I had noticed, when walking, that the sidewalk seemed to be closer than before and I wondered if something was wrong with my eyes. The problem, as it turned out, was not my eyes but my posture was stooped over at about a thirty-degree angle due to the pain and damage to the muscles.

Massage allowed me to once again walk upright. What an improvement this made to my quality of life.

I continued to go to massage every two weeks. I was getting excited that I would be able to lift weights again. Before the cancer, I prided myself on lifting weights and I could lift twenty pounds on each arm. Sadly, I had given up the thought of ever lifting weights again because of the muscle damage. Joanne told me I would be able to lift weights again. She expects my healing will continue for five more years.

Mary came to Jesus' tomb to anoint his body. He was gone. Did angels massage Jesus' broken body in the tomb? Joanne massaged my body back to life.

Dancing to Health

Kevin and I decided to return to ballroom dancing in order to help my rehabilitation. We had been taking lessons from Bob and Mary Rowswell, in London, for about four years. In the past, we took beginner's classes for about three years (we were very slow learners), then intermediate classes for one year. I nicknamed Kevin "Mr. Rigormortis" because he was so stiff when he danced. It had taken us about six months just to learn how to make a turn on the dance floor. It must have been humorous to watch us reach a wall, stop, turn our bodies, and then begin to dance again. In September 2009, we decided to go back to a beginners class because of the problems with my right arm. I needed to dance with my right hand in my pocket so as not to hurt my right arm. This actually helped Kevin become a better dancer because he became more assertive in leading the dance. Eventually, I was able to raise my right arm and do a "lady under." We attended the New Year's Eve dance organized by Bob and Mary. I managed to dance until about 10:30 p.m. when I became exhausted and we had to leave (I was certainly not Cinderella who at least got to stay out until midnight). Dancing was so much fun.

I danced in the morning when the world was young....[10]

Another Major Loss

The week before Thanksgiving, I found out my "best job in the world" would not be funded after May 14, 2010. I was devastated! I thought, *Here I am just recovering, and lo and behold I have to deal with a job loss.* I asked myself who would hire me when I have had cancer? I couldn't even work full time yet. I talked to my director, Charlene, and she cheered me up. She told me that some people see me as a survivor, not as someone whose career is over. Then I remembered that in the previous year, all I wanted to do was live for another Thanksgiving. I decided to be grateful for Thanksgiving and focus on my recovery. Luckily I had until May to find another job. I tried not ruminating, but there were many times when I felt the pain of losing the perfect job. In a paradoxical way, the thought of losing my job stopped me from thinking of myself as a victim. I had always felt reassured about the death benefits my job would provide for the family. Losing my job meant that I had to live to help them financially.

M., my cancer social worker, and I discussed how difficult it is to leave the world of cancer and return to the outside world. This is so true. In the fall, Wellspring was offering a survivor's group, and I contemplated attending. I worried, however, that I would be focused on the needs of others and not on my own recovery. I noticed I was progressively becoming more and more the nurse in my meditation group and was once again slipping into supporting others at the expense of myself. Instead, I took the opportunity to join a book club, where a group of women would discuss Sue Monk Kidd's *Dance of the Dissonant Daughter*[11]. This book describes Sue Monk Kidd's awakening in terms of what it meant to her and other women to live in a patriarchal society. The book discussed very intimate details of her spiritual journey towards recovery. I knew that patriarchy would not be my battle. My battle was to understand what I really needed and wanted from life and to learn how to rearrange my life after cancer. I read the book *Picking Up the Pieces*[12], about cancer survivors. Most of the messages I already knew; however, the stories from cancer survivors were comforting to me. They helped me to realize that I wasn't so alone in my feelings. Their stories started giving me energy to write down my thoughts and feelings for this book.

The Plague

The next big obstacle I experienced was the H1N1 flu. I don't know for sure that I contracted that particular flu virus, but I certainly had all of the symptoms. Leonie came home ill from school on the Friday before Hallowcen. Kevin was in Toronto at the annual general meeting for his work. Once again, I had to take care of Leonie while she was ill because Kevin was away. Eliza helped as much as she could. Leonie was so sick. Eliza and I both started feeling the symptoms three days later. Ironically we were supposed to be immunized the following week. I managed to hold the family together until Kevin came home the next day, but then I was very sick in bed for one week and I coughed for another five weeks. Eliza and Leonie were also home sick. Thank God Kevin worked from home for a couple of days that week. I still don't know how we balanced everything. I was so grateful that my immune system worked, but I missed Halloween again. The trick was the H1N1 virus; the treat was I survived it. We actually received the vaccine in December because it was mandatory for all health unit staff. We should now have a lifelong immunity.

What was the air like in the tomb? Was it musty? What is the fragrance of myrrh? How long does the smell of myrrh last?

November 2009

I survived to reach another birthday in November. When I was a child, everyone thought that my birthday was November 23rd, but it wasn't until I broke my arm when I was nine years old and my grandpa pulled out my birth certificate that we discovered my birthday was actually November 17th. I don't think this type of mistake happens very often when mothers are alive. To honour my youth, I decided to make a cherry chip cake because it was my favourite cake when I was a child. Making a cherry chip cake with Leonie helped me relive good memories from my childhood. I also decided to make this marshmallow-like icing that you cook on top of the stove for the cake. What a mess, and it tasted awful! We then decided to melt marshmallows and use that mixture as frosting. Another disaster occurred, but we all ate the cake with smiles on our faces. I am now going to cherish every birthday.

Mary, Joseph, the shepherds and the wise men probably didn't mix up Jesus' birthday. Mary would have reminded them.

In November, I felt the need to get to know Mona, the priest who had replaced Kate after she retired. She seemed like such a nice person, and her sermons were both spiritually uplifting and enjoyable. I started meeting with her to tell her my story. Telling Mona my story affirmed my suffering.

At the end of November, I also began noticing that I was getting progressively sadder. I thought that perhaps it was because I was so upset about losing my job or because I hadn't been sleeping well (I was up for one-and-a-half to two hours each night since July when I had stopped taking the sedative). I also wondered if the sadness was caused by decreasing levels of estrogen due to the estrogen suppressant drug I was taking to help prevent a reoccurrence of the cancer. Many women talk of mood swings, sadness, loss of energy, lack of mental concentration and focus and the inability to sleep during menopause. I thought this was the time to endure.

I told Mona of my sadness, and I started re-reading the Bible again to see if it would give me any comfort or insights. I read Genesis, and I could really see why men think that they should dominate the world. I saw sadness everywhere in the Bible. I felt very sorry for both Cain and Abel, for Isaac when he worked so long to marry Rebekah, and for Moses and for the innocent Egyptians in enduring their plagues and traumas. I really thought about the fact that so much of the Bible is about lamentations and not just one chapter. I began to wonder if the world would be a better place if we wept more.

Did Jesus weep in the tomb, or was it just his family and the disciples who wept?

On the first Sunday in Advent at the end of November, our family put up the Christmas tree. I hoped that it would bring some light into my darkness.

December 2009

The winter weather seemed to mirror my mood. The nights were getting longer, and darkness seemed to take over my days. My sadness became more pronounced, and I was crying multiple times every day. This year, with the coming of advent, I sincerely wanted to find some hope, peace, joy and love. Instead, I felt like I was drowning in sorrow. Mona organized an advent reflection that started with a shared meal. We attended as a family, and I was proud of Eliza and Leonie for contributing to the discussion. We also managed to contribute to the festivities by bringing chili and homemade macaroni and cheese one evening and gingersnap cookies on another night. On December 16th, Kevin and the girls helped decorate the Christmas tree in the sanctuary.

Even though I was feeling sad and depressed, I attended a work-related two-day retreat. It was like a funeral because I felt like it was the last time that I was ever going to have this experience. I publicly sobbed at least ten times. One of the reasons that I felt so sad was that I finally felt I had some credibility and people were listening to what I had to say. In the past, I often felt people rarely listened to or entertained my ideas.

On Christmas Eve, we travelled to my sister's house about one-and-a-half hours away. I was exhausted from the saddest December in my life, but I tried to pretend I was enjoying Christmas for the girls' sake. I knew I was a failure at that as well. I just wanted them to have a much happier Christmas than the stressful one we experienced last year. I was so relieved when Christmas was over so I would not have to pretend to be happy any longer. My friend Karen came after Christmas to visit, and it was nice. It was clear that I was depressed, but I thought that it was a situational depression (resulting from my job loss and slow recovery). I tried to convince myself that I just needed to be patient and it would eventually end, but inside, I felt like I was the damned and that no one would be able to save me.

In the middle of December, I had submitted my resume for another position at the health unit, but my heart wasn't in it. Every time I thought about the other position I started to cry. It was a good job as well; it just wasn't my job. I didn't want to leave my job until the very last minute when the research program closed.

My friends and family consistently told me to be less hard on myself, but I continued to berate myself.

This Christmas, I acted more like Herod (thinking of my own well-being) than I would have liked. I wish angels could come and tell me, "Be not afraid." I wanted to experience joy; maybe next year. Thank God Christmas comes every year, so I will have another chance. I was really glad that I could actually believe that I would be alive in another year to try again.

Was Jesus ever depressed? I bet his disciples were! How many people were sobbing on Easter Saturday? Did Jesus weep for himself? I am sure Jesus wept for the suffering of his disciples.

January 2010

In reflecting back to January 2010, I think the "darkest" point was not knowing whether or not there would be a "dawn." My crying and the depression kept getting worse and, when I interviewed for the temporary position at the health unit, I cried twice. When asked if I would commit for a year, I started to cry, thinking that all I was hoping for was to be alive in a year. Then later in the interview, I was asked what I would do after the year. Again, I started to cry, thinking *Would I be alive in one year?* Needless to say, I didn't get the job. Amazingly, I was relieved. I thought that maybe I should focus on recovery for the next few months and quit pretending that I was in any shape to apply for jobs.

We had an Epiphany lunch for our friends. It was nice to see everyone again, even though I was sad inside.

My Epiphany was that I still needed to focus on recovery and find joy, rather than looking for another job.

Mona and I continued to meet every couple of weeks, and she shared a book with me on pastoral and spiritual care. I told her how much I had thought about the Gospel of Luke and how I found it comforting.

By the middle of January, my friends were no longer gently hinting I needed to take medication. I eventually came to the conclusion I needed medication because I started obsessing about Kevin's friend who lost his wife to breast cancer about fifteen years ago. She committed suicide after her treatment was over. I knew why. I felt desperate and hopeless, but I knew I wouldn't commit suicide because I had worked in psychiatry for so long and knew the lifelong consequences to my family. Finally my obsessive suicidal thoughts made me make a doctor's appointment. I told Dr. Kumar about my crying and sadness, but I did not tell her of my suicidal thoughts. Luckily, she prescribed medication.

The first medication I took was a disaster. I became manic and couldn't sleep for three days. Colours appeared so bright they seemed psychedelic, and I had terrible abdominal pain. On the third day (I didn't notice the analogy of the time frame until right now), I went back to Dr. Kumar and told her I couldn't take it anymore. I was started on two different medications. I took one medication at night because one of its side effects was sleepiness. Dr. Kumar prescribed the second medication because of my life-long anxiety. She prescribed a week off work to see if I could get better control with the new medications without the additional stress of work.

The medication worked! I started sleeping at night right away, which made an immediate difference to my mood. It felt like a miracle. I stopped crying as frequently; I started getting the energy to work on this book; and I had more enthusiasm to work again. It is now very clear to me that I had a chemical depression (decreased levels of important chemicals in the brain and not solely a reaction to the loss of my job); otherwise I never could have recovered so quickly.

I was supposed to be back at work full time by the end of January. Our benefits insurer at work had stopped my short-term disability, because even though I had told them I was depressed, I didn't submit the medical documentation. Still, I didn't mind getting cut off from disability. It was pretty clear to me that I could only cope with a three-and-a-half-day week, so I decided to use my remaining vacation time to supplement my work week for the remaining four-teen weeks of work. I took every Wednesday and most Friday mornings off so I could go to meditation. This was such a good idea, and I really started to feel better. While I was working during my treatment, I often felt guilty for not working harder; now I felt relieved to have the days off. I even gained some pleasure from them.

I was also beginning to become more aware that some aspects of healing were occurring so gradually that I hadn't really noticed them before. During my treatment, I never felt well enough to drive. It was like Kevin (or someone else) was "Driving Miss Pat," similar to the movie "Driving Miss Daisy." After the treatment was over, I was frightened to drive. Everything about driving seemed overwhelming. I had begun driving again the previous June, but parking lots were overwhelming. Cars seemed to come out of nowhere. I would park at the very back, away from other cars. It seemed as though there were jaywalkers everywhere that could or would step out onto the road in front of me. I knew I needed to become more independent, so I began driving to meditation. To be extra cautious, however, I would take the back routes and I would not parallel park. I drove slower than the speed limit and would sometimes get very nasty looks from other drivers. Then slowly, almost imperceptibly, I started to feel less agitated while driving. It seemed like I was becoming more aware of my environment so it wasn't as frightening. I started taking main roads again. Driving after dark is still challenging, but I now believe that it will get better after my energy levels improve a bit more.

My sessions at meditation continued to be healing. I was persistently getting two messages: I still had work to complete, and I needed to learn to take better care of myself. I understood that dancing lessons, meditation and Sunday church services all gave me a sense of hope and rejuvenation, but I knew that I needed more than four hours of rejuvenation a week to recover.

Towards the end of January, I told my meditation group that Kevin always postpones the New Year until February 1st. His reasoning was that we shouldn't start a new year paying for the Christmas and New Year celebrations. This led to a discussion about St. Brigid's Day (a Celtic saint). Deborah, our meditation leader, mentioned that February 1st is celebrated because the seeds of spring are present before we see the results. We then had a guided meditation to a garden. I was surprised to visualize the Garden of Eden. There was a stag with the most majestic antlers and the deepest, wisest, kindest eyes accompanying me through the garden. This led me to think about the seeds of recovery being present before you can see the results. I was talking about this the following week, and Deborah told me that St. Brigid was the saint of healing. I decided the period of lamentation might be ending. I was grateful for the antidepressants that brought me out of the depths of despair and enabled me to once again feel hopeful. I even wondered if I had suffered with the depression so I could tell people about this experience. I now really understand how people with a chronic illness can become exhausted over time and experience a chemical depression. It is really easy to understand how people can feel hopeless enough to have suicidal thoughts. Thank God there was help available.

I continued to focus on my physical, emotional and spiritual healing and had a surge of hope when I passed another oncology visit at the beginning of February. I became more determined to start ridding myself of some of my fears. My increased energy levels then helped contribute to a compulsive urge to work on this book. My creativity was coming back, and the words just flowed from my fingers. Kate read the first draft out loud to me and thought it was very good. Kate's praise meant a lot to me, and it gave me more confidence my book could make a difference to the lives of other families in similar situations.

On Valentine's Day, Kevin and I decided to go to the dance sponsored by our dance instructors, Bob and Mary. I was looking forward to it. The day of the dance I made a very big decision. I decided to shave my legs. It's funny, but watching the hair grow back on my legs had been a source of comfort after losing it for about nine months. Up until then, I had no desire to shave my legs even though I had friction burn every time my legs happened to rub together.

Maybe this is how it feels when you start to take off the shroud.

The terrible black circles under my eyes started to recede very slowly as I slept more. At the Valentine's dance, I saw someone I hadn't seen since I was sick. I explained what had happened to me without crying or even feeling sad. She told me that I was really looking good and she would not have known I was sick if I hadn't told her. The next day at church was Transfiguration Sunday. I thought about how Jesus' face shone when talking to Elijah and Moses on the mountain and how my eyes now occasionally had a shine.

Maybe, like Jesus during the transfiguration or like Abraham Maslow (who investigated peak moments of self-

actualizing people[13]), I was beginning to have a "mountain experience." The days were getting longer and brighter. I felt like light was coming back into my world after a long period of darkness. I told myself that by Easter Sunday my nine-month period of Easter Saturday would be over. I would come out from the tomb and go forward. I was going to celebrate the Easter season and finish my book by Pentecost Sunday. I thought it was an amazing coincidence that the period of Easter season coincided with my last radiation treatment on May 22, 2009.

In order to achieve my goal, I made a commitment to myself to use the time between then and Easter to learn what it means to rejuvenate and to take care of myself. For months in metta meditation, I was saying the following phrases:

> May I feel God's love and learn to love and take care
> of myself;
> May I be a survivor and feel joy;
> May I listen to God's word and be open;

Now I added:

> May I find ways to re-energize.

It was beginning to feel like Saturday evening in the tomb. I wonder if Jesus realized on Saturday night that he would shortly be going back into the world.

On Ash Wednesday, I decided to focus on understanding how Jesus was able to re-energize and persevere in the wilderness so he could go forward with his mission. I didn't think that a paradigm of suffering would benefit me. I had already experienced too much suffering.

Earlier in the book, I talked about dreams that provided comfort to me, but I also think it is important to listen to nightmares as well. When I was young, I would often dream about tsunamis. I would be on the shore and see a humongous wave coming towards me. Before I knew it, I would be submerged under the water, frantically trying to swim, and then I would awake. These nightmares mirrored my feelings of inadequacy and being overwhelmed as a youth. Years later, I would have recurring dreams about not completing my course work for school, and they continued right through my studies for my PhD. I dreamt that the semester at school was almost over, but I did not know the teacher or professor and they did not know me. I felt desperate because I knew I would not graduate if I did not hand in the assignments.

Ten years ago, I had five miscarriages over a two year period, before we adopted Leonie. The night before one of my miscarriages, I remember dreaming that I was walking along the street and fell into a pothole. I awoke convinced something bad would happen and it did. I had another miscarriage. Since the time of my miscarriages, I would often dream that I was pregnant and something bad would happen. One night in March 2010, I dreamt that my niece had a successful pregnancy. Later in the dream, I was also pregnant. All of a sudden, as I was standing by the sink in the kitchen, the membranes broke and amniotic fluid came flowing out, but I didn't go into labour. I was very frightened because I didn't even feel the baby moving and I was convinced the baby was dead. I told people, but no one seemed to notice or care.

Dreams can really tell us important information about how we are feeling. This dream mirrored my disturbing feelings of complete powerlessness, feeling like no one noticed or cared about me, just like when I was a child. I knew I was healing because I didn't feel as powerless as often, although the feelings still lurked somewhere deep in the recesses of my brain. Even though a dream can point to feelings of powerlessness, my ability to respond in life was not disabled. A couple of days after the last disturbing dream, I updated my resume and cover letter and applied for a job. I also started to think about clothing.

The Girls

In the middle of February, Ruth, a friend of mine who had previously had a double mastectomy sixteen years ago, asked if I wanted to go with her to buy a new prosthesis and bras. I knew I had no desire to wear a bra ever again, but I wanted to go along to find out what it was like. We met at the prosthesis store, and I must admit I felt emotionally and physically uncomfortable. The muscles and fascia (membranes over the muscles) in my right chest area were still sore, so that I would be unable to try on any bras. Just looking at the bras made me realize how uncomfortable they would be given the flaps under my arms where the drains from the surgery were inserted. Yikes! My biggest surprise was the language in the world of prostheses. The sales lady called the prostheses *the girls*. Up until this point, I had always thought of the girls only as Eliza and Leonie. Apparently there is also a more advanced prosthesis available so you don't sweat under it. Picking the right bra for Ruth was a difficult process. There were pretty bras and "leisure" bras that looked terrible but feel comfortable. Even though there are government supplements to assist in paying for these prostheses and bras, the cost of prostheses and bras seems like highway robbery to me. I think it is a terrible injustice that women who undergo such trauma should also be subjected to such high costs, just to try and look "feminine" or conform to society's version of "normal." I left the store feeling exhausted and more committed to my idea of starting a line of clothing that incorporates a place to put in a light prosthesis (so I don't have a caved-in look). I absolutely do not want a bra rubbing against those flaps!

In March, I started to discuss with Eliza her tardiness in writing her section for this book. Since she was currently taking grade nine English and needed to write a speech each week, we agreed she could use some of her speeches for my book because, as she says, "Don't you know I have a lot of homework?"

Eliza is a beautiful writer and often expresses her feelings in her writing. Last year when she was in grade eight, she inevitably killed off the hero in all of her stories. I remember one story that Eliza wrote quite poignantly. Eliza and I were on a boat trip and a terrible storm came out of the blue. It was clear that the boat was going to sink. Eliza and I huddled together and told each other how much we love each other and then the boat sank. We could see each other submerged under the water, and we were reaching out for each other. Eliza felt safe and comforted when angels came and took us away.

Certainly this story was about Eliza's fear of me dying. My tears actually flowed again as I thought about this story. I hate to see my children suffer. I hate to see myself suffer. I interpreted this story as the cancer being the bad storm. The boat sinking meant that we both died, meaning life was over for her as well. *No one walked on the water.* Nevertheless, Eliza knows there are some comforts in life because angels came to help her. Eliza wrote many stories that year with similar themes; she vented her fears and anxieties through her writing.

It is interesting that Eliza needed to write a speech on personal power in grade nine English, just when I was wondering where I would get my energy and how Jesus got energy in the wilderness. I was so proud of her that she could reflect on her life as she did.

Eliza's stories describe how she has matured through our crisis. Her story "Invincible" (found at the end of chapter one) shows the loss of some of her naiveté. Her cherished moment just happened to be one of my cherished moments. I wish that I could have had her ability to write "My Personal Power" at the age of fourteen years. Eliza was learning to balance fear and hope, something I was still learning, only forty years later. When I reflect on my personal power, I knew attending church, my dance lessons with Kevin, quietly curling up with Eliza and Leonie in my nice warm bed, going for my daily walks and meditation were the things that helped me.

Personal Power
By Eliza

I get the strength and will to continue through the journey of life with the power I receive from my family and friends, creativity, and by the magical worlds of books.

I get power from my family and friends because they're always there when I'm sad, scared, or just need someone. Even though my sister and I fight constantly and are opposites from one another, I know that if I need her she would put her differences aside and be there for me. If I'm sad my friends are there to make me laugh and bring joy back into to my life. My parents are understanding and caring and would always support me even if my decisions are not the best. I can trust my family and friends to keep me safe, that's why they're my power.

Creativity brings me power because when I'm doing my art I feel safe as if I belong and it helps me truly express myself in ways words cannot. Art helps me deal with my emotions instead of bottling them up. When I'm doing art I'm focused and I let go of my worries and just feel what I want to feel. Art is truly magical. It creates beauty out of nothing and it feels like I give my artwork part of my soul so it can show the emotion within it. That's why creativity is my power.

Books are my power because when I'm not feeling happy I can pick up a book and escape into a magical world where anything is possible. I can leave my worries and fears behind and take the role of a character and their emotions. I can be anything and have an adventure of a life time, that's why books are my power.

I can always count on my family and friends to be here and keep me safe; they are my power. Creativity brings me joy and lets me express myself; creativity is my power. Books transport me to a magical world where I can have an adventure of a life time; books are my power. With friends, family, creativity and books in my life, I will always have the power to be myself.

My Most Cherished Moment

By Eliza

I still remember like it was yesterday, the moment in life where I was truly happy and peaceful. I was at a cottage near Ottawa; it was the first, but not last time I went there.

I was sitting on a comfy swing that gently rocked back and forth. The last of the fiery setting sun shot colors of red, orange, yellow and purple into the sky. The stars were just starting to twinkle. The sky's colors were reflected in the calm shimmering water beneath. The cool breeze kissed my cheeks and danced with the bright green leaves. A fish rippled the otherwise still surface of the water. I can still smell the wonderful aroma of fresh damp grass that surrounded the trees and lanes nearby. The sweet flavour of homemade strawberry ice cream exploded in my mouth.

My dad was telling one of his lame jokes again while my little sister ran around the deck to the lake trying to catch a frog. The sound of my mother's laughter filled the silence. Everything was as it should be, calm and relaxed with no worries.

This memory always brings a smile to my face; it will be in my heart and soul forever.

My weekly meditation continued to be a source of inspiration and hope for me. The guided imagery of meditation, however, started to become a surreal experience. As mentioned earlier, I thought my subconscious and God were comforting me and providing direction. I had experienced one meditation with the majestic stag in the Garden of Eden, but that didn't feel right as the power animal Deborah (our meditation leader) described. (Power animals were real or mythic animals that give people energy, similar to totems in aboriginal cultures.) I felt good about the visualization of the stag, but it still didn't seem to fit as my personal totem. I have previously mentioned the hymn "On Eagle's Wings" that has always resonated with me and brought me comfort. In past meditation sessions, a very large eagle would come to welcome me and I would climb on its back and, flying very fast, it would take me high into the clouds. During this meditation, I realized that the eagle was my totem source of power; so I began meditating about this eagle. It was so big in my mind's eye that it could block out the sun. This eagle felt like it had been around since the beginning of the world. When I touched it, I felt powerful myself.

In a recent meditation, we were to go into a cave and meet an "old wise one." This incredibly large eagle miraculously shrunk so it could sit on my shoulder as we entered the cave. The "old one" bowed to the eagle, indicating it was the higher power. The old one told me I was to still try and find ways to reenergize because there was work that I had to do after I healed. What remarkable and hopeful imagery. I know in my heart that my "eagle" and God are related; I am just not sure how. Now when Deborah asks us at the beginning of the mediation to imagine a time when we felt peaceful and strong, I visualize my eagle companion and let the eagle take care of me. It is funny though, as hard as I try to visualize it, I cannot tell if the eagle is male or female.

In writing this book, I have had many feelings of trepidation about my self-exposure. In some ways, identifying myself as a Christian was harder for me than pouring out the physical health issues and describing the emotional suffering that we, as a family, experienced. I have always gone to church but rarely disclosed my beliefs to anyone outside the church. Now it felt like the whole world was going to know about my religious and spiritual life. Luckily Dr. Potvin referred me to Helen, the spiritual care counsellor at the cancer clinic, to help me through the next stage of my recovery. I arrived feeling worried and guilty because I parked the car in a shopping mall parking lot that had signs indicating that unauthorized vehicles would get towed. When I entered her office, the first thing I did was "confess" about the car. Helen told me they do indeed tow, so I ran out and moved my car to another parking lot. I haven't done much running over the last eighteen months, so I was winded when I returned. Amazingly, it was still a very fruitful thirty minutes. I explained my goals around Lent and told her how important communion was to me during the illness. Helen was willing to talk to me about my experience and this book. She was very interested in my analogies about Jesus' passion, especially concerning Easter Saturday. She *lent* (no pun intended) me a book on the fullness of communion even though we had not discussed how I treated chemo like communion.[14] She also lent me *Bone* by Marion Woodman.[15] I talked to her about my fears of exposure in writing this book within a spirituality theme, even though I felt like it was my "responsibility" to write this story. She asked me a question that still makes me feel uncomfortable. She asked me how I would feel to become "known." We always talk about God "fully" knowing us, but I feel anxious with the thought that complete strangers will "know" intimate details about me and my family. I left feeling like Helen came into my life so that I could finish up the last stages of this book.

We had our second annual bean soup party on February 27, 2008. It was so nice to have the people who drove me to radiation come together, even though two couples were ill and unable to attend. It was a splendid night. The one thing I would like to mention is my preference for hearing success stories about people who have battled cancer and survived. These stories help me believe I can also survive. At the party, someone I love dearly told me about a woman she knew who had breast cancer three years ago. This woman was recently diagnosed with cancer of the eye. When I heard this news, I was completely overwhelmed. My sinus had been hurting just a little bit for about a week and my vision was a little blurry in my right eye. I automatically believed that I had eye cancer and needed chemo again. I was so disappointed to hear this news when I was having such a lovely evening that I immediately crashed emotionally. I quietly left the room to try and compose myself. I called Kevin over and told him what happened and asked him the big question: "Do you think that I have eye cancer?" He smiled and said "no" but he agreed to come with me to get my eyes checked. That night, he lay down with me for awhile before I went to sleep. In the morning I felt better. I could now say a prayer for the woman who had to face cancer treatment once again.

I just know that Jesus would not have been consumed with worry for himself if he heard the story of someone else's suffering. He would have helped. I knew I was still in the wilderness, fearing the wild beasts would destroy me. Would I ever have enough faith to be able to feel safe in the wilderness? I was glad that by morning I could say a prayer for the woman undergoing chemo.

I continued to discover other small signs of healing. Last summer, the enamel on my front teeth appeared translucent. I had been taking a calcium supplement since last June 2009, when I discovered that I had minimal osteoporosis. By March 2010, my teeth had lost most of their translucency and were looking healthier.

I also heard that one of my manuscripts was getting published. I had been successful in publishing papers over the past eighteen months, but this one was different. It was an extension of my dissertation. My PhD advisor was adamant that I try and publish it by myself (no co-authors). I was reluctant to do this since I have always involved others in my papers. The paper went for peer review in December, 2008, but when I did not hear whether they would accept it, I contacted the journal in November 2009. Then I started checking my email a few times every day in anticipation of hearing a decision, but, there was no word. I contacted the publisher again in February, even though I felt hesitant because I didn't want to appear "pushy." I found out in March that this paper was going to be published. The publisher did not even ask for any revisions. This paper is significant because it reflects that even when I was in limbo (the tomb) and feeling passive, something good like a publication could still happen. I viewed this as another signal that it was time to prepare for my exit from the tomb.

March 6th, 2009, was the first anniversary of the mastectomy surgery. I was in a meeting at the health unit when the hour came. I had been watching the clock tick by minute by minute towards the time of surgery; this time I wasn't anesthetized and I didn't have to fear scalpels. My arm and shoulder were sore, but not from surgery. I had fallen two days before and landed on my right arm, pushing it into my body. I worried I might get lymphodema, but it didn't swell. I remembered that I would be going to Joanne, my massage therapist, the following Wednesday, and I had confidence that she would "fix" it. Lots of things were starting to feel "fixed."

In December 2009, I began reading Carl Jung's biography[16]. I was reading it because I knew Jung went on a journey of personal discovery and analyzed his dreams and visions to discover their meaning. I was hoping that reading his biography would give me some insight into my own experiences. One passage in particular made me smile. Jung said it was a good thing for people to be neurotic because neurotic people were unlikely to be delusional. I wondered whether there were any Jungian symbols (archetypes) surrounding cancer? There are definitely archetypes surrounding suffering and feeling like a victim such as the phoenix. *Where is my phoenix?*

I have wanted Kevin to read some of my work for many, many years; so much so that I often harboured resentment towards him. This is because when we were first married, I constantly edited his work when he started university as a mature student to get his degree in history. In the past, he would always tell me he was inadequate to read my work. I still harboured resentment. In March, he began reading the first draft of this book. I am very grateful, even though I noticed I was feeling inadequate because he found *so* many edits. Kevin also said something that surprised me. He said, "I sound like a jerk!" I could tell that his feelings were hurt, but I wasn't sure how much.

I asked him why he felt like a jerk, and he mentioned the times he had to go away when I was ill. During those periods, the girls were usually ill or stressed, thereby increasing my burden. I have mentioned throughout this book my issues with abandonment, and to tell the truth, I did feel abandoned and probably resentful toward him. "Isn't it enough to deal with cancer, without carrying all of the family problems as well?"

The big question at the moment became "Is Kevin a jerk?" In response, I would like to say that Kevin has been there for me many times over the almost twenty years of our relationship, first as a friend, then as my husband and the father of my children. He has been there the vast amount of time when I have been neurotic, and I don't think that he has ever felt that I was less of a person for my neuroses. In the beginning of our marriage, he was striving to be successful at university and then in his career. He was a late starter, but I admired him for his willingness to change. His biggest challenge was always his lack of confidence. Twenty years ago, a stranger would hear his stutter and see his inability to take charge of situations. Now, he is much more self-confident, doesn't stutter and has a responsible position at work. He is still a kind and thoughtful person and admired by everyone I know, often receiving nominations for sainthood because he is married to *me*! He was the nicest man I knew twenty years ago, and nothing has changed.

What then was the dilemma? I think the problem was that I wanted to know he admired me and, after all of the early abandonment issues I faced, I wanted to know he would be there for me when I needed him. It was very easy for me to manage all of the strategic decisions for the family (finances, parenthood issues, being social), and Kevin just let me do it. I always felt responsible for the family's overall emotions, including Kevin's, but no one seemed particularly interested in supporting mine. This did not become an issue until I "fell down" because of my illness. My illness was clearly bigger than cancer because I had to deal with many interpersonal issues as well. I also wanted Kevin to transition into a leadership and protective role, just when he was stressed to the max.

My friends tell me I am their hero. Kevin tells me I am brimming over with courage. In fact, I know most people see me as courageous. One of the big problems in my relationship with Kevin was that I did not see myself as a hero. I would continue to say that there is a big difference between functioning under stress and how you feel about yourself. People would say I am a hero, and I think they say that because they want me to know that they admire me. I would often feel frustrated, however, because I thought they were not acknowledging my distress. There is a very big gap between these responses.

Jesus was clearly the hero of the New Testament. I wonder if he felt like a hero or that he was just doing God's work. I wonder if his disciples felt like jerks. I imagine if the disciples reviewed their track record prior to Jesus' crucifixion, they would not think their behaviour was stellar. What did that parable mean again? Who comes first? Who is the best? Maybe we all need to go through the self-reflection of "Am I a jerk?" before we can really move on to discovering what is important in life.

Is Kevin a jerk? No, he is not a jerk. Is there room for our marriage to get better? Absolutely. Has he grown through our family's experience of cancer? Absolutely. I think he has moved beyond many of his adolescent insecurities as shown by his interactions with our older daughter, Eliza. He is beginning to see he has something to offer Eliza as he assists her with her homework in geography. He is starting to hang out with his children and ask them how they are and about their day. I am immensely grateful for these changes.

What would it take for Kevin to become my hero? I don't know if it is surprising that I primarily want him to act like he wants to be with me; that he enjoys my company; that he can communicate to me that he is proud of my achievements. I want him to notice the things I have done for him and for the girls. It became evident that Kevin was feeling better because is much more helpful in preparing meals, cleaning up the house and spending time with the girls. I don't need a hero to save me. God is the only one who can save me, and I think for the moment (I still need qualifiers) I am doing okay. The safety I need from Kevin is mainly telling me he still wants to be with me. This is the message I want from my type of hero.

The Robin-Orange-Breast Birds Are Returning

On March 25, 2010, I could tell the first days of spring had arrived. I was up in my bed recovering from a bad cold, and to my surprise, I saw a robin-orange-breast bird in the tree outside my bedroom window. I have retold this story at least a thousand times, but I am going to retell it again because it really reflects how I looked at the world and what I consider injustice. When I was in kindergarten, we had to colour a picture of the "robin-red-breast." It was probably a surprise test on "colours," but every robin in southwestern

Ontario had an orange breast. So of course, I coloured it orange. The little kid next to me coloured his or her picture of the breast orange as well. My teacher, Mrs. W. came by and got angry because the robin's breast was coloured orange. The child beside me told the teacher that he or she did it because of me. Instead of seeing me as a budding environmentalist, Mrs. W. was angry and sent me to the corner for what felt like an eternity. I thought the crime of "copying" should have been acknowledged because I was right about the colour. I didn't make the other child "copy" me. No, I was the only person sent to the corner. I thought this was a major injustice then, and I still do. The crime was blindness on the teacher's part for being rigid and unkind and for not explaining there can be a difference between primary colours and birds. She shamed me in front of the whole kindergarten class. She shamed me many times in front of the kindergarten class. When your mom dies and you are shamed in front of the class, you remember. It starts a process of dismembering your self-worth, and there is no one to "kiss it better" when you go home.

As the season of Lent was coming to a close, I was struggling to decide if I was actually ready to come out of the tomb on Easter Sunday. It is very clear in my mind that Easter Saturday is not just twenty-four hours. It is like the idea of God creating the world in seven literal days. Easter Saturday had already spanned nine months, as long as the gestation period of a pregnancy.

During March break I had a setback with worrying when we were away on a holiday. I became frantic for what now seems like a minor reason. Instead of accepting that it was unfortunate and just move on, I proceeded to once again "beat myself up," berating myself for being completely neurotic and for questioning whether I could ever change. Then I got a head cold, which made me feel physically ill and not just emotionally ill. I became sullen and fretful. My behaviour wrecked the end of my vacation when I was really looking forward to getting away. How was someone so eternally neurotic ever going to be able to feel the resurrection of Easter?

When I began to calm down, I decided that maybe I needed to define what *resurrection* would mean for me. In my reflections, I decided to no longer "be anxious about being anxious." I have been anxious since I was a child and always afraid that something would happen expectedly or unexpectedly, causing me to die. Even as a child, I learned to keep these fears and anxieties hidden as "dirty secrets" It was clear to me, even then, that people consider someone, regardless of their age, as unworthy and unattractive for possessing these personality flaws. I became very good at publicly hiding my anxiety. I hid these anxieties and fears from everyone but my trusted friends. I don't know if it was fortunate or unfortunate the cancer had depleted me so much that I could no longer hide the anxieties and fears. I berated myself even more because now everyone knew about my anxieties and fears. In my reflections, I realized many of my caretakers did find me neurotic, but I was not aware of them seeing me as less worthy. I realized I wasn't going to die from anxiety, but my fears and anxieties were depleting my quality of life. I therefore started counting some positives in my life to counteract some of the many negative thoughts and memories. During my horrific experience of treatment and recovery, I did manage to leave behind my past anger and resentments. I truly do not have an underlying anger anymore. I also managed to leave most of my anaphylaxis phobias behind since I now considered them a "luxury item." I stopped thinking of death every day, considering it another luxury item that I couldn't afford. Maybe I could take the next step of stopping the negative voice saying I am unworthy because of the anxieties and fears.

I then started a series of confessions and asked for help. I made an appointment with my family doctor (Dr. Kumar) and I told her about "being anxious about being anxious" and I wanted to stop this behaviour. I asked if I could come in when I felt anxious to discuss my fears. (For example, is the pimple by my incision line that hasn't healed in three weeks cancerous?) She was very compassionate with me, and we agreed I would come in regularly to go over my fears of the cancer returning without "shame." I met with Deborah, my meditation leader, and confessed my strange experiences during meditation. She reassured me the comforting voices that I heard did not mean I was going "crazy." She said, "They are a gift." I confessed to Helen, the pastoral care leader at the cancer clinic, about the "shames" of my life. She suggested that maybe I could create a ritual "to lay these shames at the cross" to further my healing; a solution I could relate to within a Christian paradigm.

I created this ritual on Good Friday, 2010. I asked Kate to come with me as I re-walked the labyrinth at Medaille House. During the process of walking into the centre of the labyrinth, I thought about everything that had made me sad, angry, resentful and shamed. First, I thought about the loss of my mother and about being friendless and neglected when I was young. I thought about the death of my grandfather and about how I was bullied when I had no one to protect me. I thought about my struggles with a learning disability and about the miscarriages. To my surprise, I had managed to get almost to the centre of the labyrinth before I thought about the cancer. By that point, cancer didn't seem to have the same significance as it did even thirty minutes before. In the centre of the labyrinth, I lit a candle and Kate blessed a cross that I had made using bamboo and my old bra strap. I left my shame in the centre of the labyrinth. On the way out of the labyrinth, I thought about the things for which I am grateful. I would keep my new cross as a reminder in case I fell back into the old ways of berating myself for being anxious.

Did Jesus ever feel shame? He was always so confident. Don't you know that I was in my father's house? He could sleep during the storm on Lake Galilee when all of the disciples feared that they were going to drown. Peter felt terrible shame when he denied Jesus three times after being so "cocky" about not doing it. Are you really ever human until you have felt shame? I don't know if Jesus personally felt shame, but Helen and Kate assure me that he took our shames and left them on the cross. That is our resurrection.

During a recent sermon, Alistair, a New Testament professor, explained that the word *prodigal* means "extravagant." My anxiety was my extravagance. Tanya, a friend from mediation, said, "When you grow up in a neurotic environment, you end up neurotic." Kate said my anxiety is a physiological condition. "Do diabetics lack faith because they are not healed?" Extravagance can be forgiven, whether it is intentional or unintentional. Kate once mentioned, "You can't have peace without truth." My truth is that I am an anxious person. I may always be an anxious person. Maybe as time goes on, I will be able to relax and be less of an anxious person. My anxiety, though, does not make me unworthy, just human. Every time I do something to help Eliza and Leonie, I am also helping my lonely inner child to heal. I do kiss things better when they come home hurt and afraid. I do help them learn to cope and find some pleasures in life.

I had been very anxious about a pimple that was located close to my incision line and had not healed in over four weeks. I remembered that Dr. Pereira said cancer cells can hide in the skin. Kate mentioned a speaker she had heard on the radio and suggested using her technique. This woman spoke of "truth" to help cope with anxiety.

Question: Is my pimple cancer?

Answer: I don't know.

Question: Do I absolutely know if my pimple is cancer?

Answer: No.

Question: How do I feel when I think my pimple is cancer?

Answer: I am tearful and weepy. I am afraid of having chemo and radiation again. I feel helpless and hopeless.

Question: How would I feel if it wasn't true?

Answer: I didn't have an answer.

I have been anxious for most of my life. With a little prodding, Kate suggested I might feel happy and relieved.[17] I think Kate helped me achieve another "epiphany." Maybe I am ready to ask the questions of truth. "You can't have peace without truth." Kate also said, "Who said peace isn't work?"

On Easter Saturday night, Kevin and I attended the Easter Vigil at the Anglican cathedral to mark the end of my period in Easter Saturday. This was the first time we had ever attended an Easter Vigil. It was a beautiful service. At the beginning of the service, a paschal candle was lit to remember Jesus' resurrection. Then in the darkness of the sanctuary, everyone lit individual candles to share the light. I know I am not alone in having fears that the cancer will return. I will continue to have anxieties and need support as I try to cope. Nevertheless, this is not a good enough reason to stay in the tomb. The paschal candle means there is still time for healing.

Reflections:

- I was physically, emotionally, and spiritually exhausted after the treatment was completed. I experienced post-traumatic stress as a result of my treatment and needed time to heal in the tomb.
- The hormone treatment perhaps should be spelled "hor-moan" because it removed the defences that I created to hide my emotions. Dropping levels of estrogen were saving my life, but the price was tears, forgetfulness, irritability and sleep deprivation.
- The fatigue from radiation therapy was like none other I have ever known. Did Sleeping Beauty and Rip Van Winkle have cancer treatment before they slept for 20 or 100 years?
- Was Jesus really in the tomb for only one day?
- Massage therapy was critical to my well-being. Muscle contractures are a sign of terrible damage. Each ounce of pain during massage was worth it to allow me to have full range of motion of my right arm, to stand tall

again instead of being stooped over and to breathe or bend over without pain.

- I had to let go of the anger I had when my family could not put my needs ahead of their own. The only solution was to forgive and begin again.
- Counsellors can easily tell spouses to come "out of the back of the cave" and send the ill person to the back of the cave for rest. It is not so easy to do!
- Family therapy really helped the girls to move into Easter way ahead of Kevin and myself.
- Sister C. really affirmed me when she said that it was a miracle I survived my treatment. God would take care of me and send help. Help came.
- My expectations of myself are much too high. It would have been better if I believed that I deserved to weep, sob and moan. My depression under the circumstances was natural.
- Depression can be treated. I should have sought treatment before I became obsessed with suicidal thoughts. The symptoms were primarily over within two weeks after starting the medication.
- I should have reached out for more help. My friends wanted to help. I should have realized I wouldn't have been a burden on them.
- The signs of healing are often present before they are recognized.
- Regular meditation helped me connect better with God and to heal.
- The fear of dying may take a long time to recede.
- It is difficult to leave the world of cancer and try to function with whatever people call the "new normal."

- On Easter Saturday, we should all wear the "black bands of grieving" from olden times. They symbolize "Be gentle with us."
- Please tell success stories. It is easy to worry that when cancer comes back to someone else you could be next. I cognitively know cancer can return and be successfully treated again. It is just that I don't have the faith to believe it yet. I don't know if I have the stamina to know how I could cope if something serious does happen.
- Knowing that you want to take off the shroud is a sign that healing is progressing well.
- Leave your shame at the cross. You can't truly heal when you feel shame.
- Accepting yourself and finding peace can be hard work.
- Easter Saturday ends when you can see the light because the boulder blocking the front of the tomb is miraculously gone.

Chapter 10

A Journey with Pat Sealy
Rev. Kate Hathaway

Pat is a nurse with a PhD in sociology, married with two daughters aged fourteen and ten. She and I met many years ago through Dundas Street United Church, where she and her husband Kevin and my husband Alistair attended. We did not socialize often over the years, but shortly before Pat's diagnosis we had reconnected at dinner parties with two other couples. My initial feeling when Pat was diagnosed with advanced breast cancer was of concern for her and her family. I was also dismayed that her health care providers had not diagnosed her illness earlier when she first sought help. My next thought was, "Here we go again—another vibrant woman with breast cancer."

Like many women of my age, I have walked this road before with friends or family members, some of whom are alive and, well, some of whom are not. Unlike many women of my age, I have been a hospital chaplain and was assigned in my initial training to leukemia patients, and it is my experience that ministry with the seriously ill is where I have been most dramatically aware of the presence of Holy Spirit.

So as I embarked on this journey with Pat, I trusted that Holy Spirit would be present and guide us.

Pat was devastated by her diagnosis (who wouldn't be?), but her major worry was that history was going to repeat itself and that, like her mother, she was going to die young and leave her children orphaned. If there was a positive side to this anxiety, it was that she was determined to do everything she needed to do to get better, despite her fears and apprehensions. There was no choice in her mind about whether or not to have chemotherapy, surgery and radiation—she just had to get on with it. And so she began to strategize and organize; scheduling appointments, visits, meals, rides, breaks, counselling, child minding—everything she and her family needed to get through this gruelling journey. And she began to attend the little Anglican church close by where I was the priest. I visited her in her home to give her the space to listen to her own voice, her fear of dying, her fear of infection and her own processing of the gruelling treatments she was receiving. The treatments and the trauma were causing her to reassess her life and shifting her priorities as they diminished her capacity to function as she had before. Pat felt uncomfortable leaving the safe haven of her home but wanted to socialize, so Ali and I were often invited over for dinner with the family.

The Chaplain's Perspective

Because Pat had been abandoned as a child by her father and by her mother's death and then by her grandparent's death, she could not trust the world to provide what she needed or trust people to stick around. Her primary attachments had systematically disappeared, and consequently she suffered from acute anxiety, which she masked under a cloak of competency. As a result of having no one but herself to rely on, she had become very resourceful. She is a pragmatist, good at managing, articulating what needs to be done and getting it done. This looks like control, but is actually a survival technique. Pat has had more than her fair share of challenges in life, and we talked about these and about how her illness had given her the opportunity to confront some unresolved issues. We also talked about how having experienced deprivation and loss, she has deep understanding of suffering and has carved out an identity for herself as caregiver. As we processed some of her history, she became aware that she probably over functions, taking care of others at the expense of herself. She began to see her illness as giving her an opportunity to reflect and to pray.

Prayer

What prayer is not. It is not about getting God to change Her mind. I do not believe God sends illness. God does not send illness, but it seems that illness is one of the things that slow us down enough to acknowledge that *God is.* It has been said that in our fast-paced, work-oriented Western culture, illness provides the only legitimate opportunity to meditate. Prayer, our conversations with God, our listening to God, our ranting at God, our stillness with God, can bring us healing. It does not always bring cure, but it does bring healing. Prayer is not about magic, and I totally reject the idea that if you don't get what you want you didn't pray hard enough or that God picks and chooses who will be healed and who will not. Prayer and healing and how it works are a mystery. Pat prayed a lot. She prayed for others, and others prayed for her. How good it is when we pray and when, if only for a moment, we stop to recognize that someone somewhere is praying for us.

The Eucharist: *an outward and visible sign of an inward and spiritual grace.*

Eucharist is central to my faith journey and to my practice of ministry. As coordinator of pastoral services at University Hospital, I celebrated Holy Communion regularly in the sanctuary on the main floor of the hospital. The service would be announced on the overhead speakers throughout the hospital, and staff who could not attend would comment that even though they could not attend, they felt comforted when they heard the announcement. Often I would take communion to the bedside of patients. As a student, I remember what a privilege it was to take the sacrament to a young leukemia patient whom I had attended for several months. He was in isolation after a bone marrow transplant and could only manage to consume half of the tiny wafer because his mouth was so sore from chemotherapy, but through the communion wafer (the host), which had been sanctified at a local church, he became part of the wider community; he was no longer in isolation. Jesus was indeed present in that hospital room, and it was one of the few times this stoic nineteen year old allowed himself to cry.

Prior to Pat's surgery, I took communion to her home. I celebrated in the quiet of her living room and afterwards gave her a blessing with the laying on of hands. "Our Lord Jesus and His disciples laid hands upon the sick…pray that as we follow His example, you may know the power of his unfailing love." She said she felt comforted and strengthened.

My Own Journey

When reflecting with a fellow traveller, one cannot help but reflect on one's own story, and I found myself becoming aware that I too have become better at taking care of others than myself, and that we must pay attention to ourselves if we are to take good care of others. I have spent my working life in the role of caregiver as a teacher, parent, in hospitals and in the parish. In early 2009, I began to experience some minor health issues, which I read as a reminder to slow down. Also, two of my offspring were about to give birth, providing Ali and me with a total of seven grandchildren, and I wanted to have the luxury of spending time with them. As a consequence of all this, I made a very healthy decision: I was going to retire. I had done some writing during my chaplaincy years and continue to write poetry and prose. I have visions of publishing but have never found the time to edit and organize.

Jesus said that it is in giving that we receive. Often we give because of our own need, and while there is merit in that, giving can become pathological—in the sense that it can be unhealthy. The insights I gained on my journey with Pat may or may not have helped her, but I suspect there has been some spiritual healing for both of us, because God is good and kind and loving and patient and there is amazing grace. And curiously, here am I, the "would be" author, writing a chapter in Pat's book, and she is healed. God does indeed move in mysterious ways Her wonders to perform.

Chapter 11

Easter Sunday Reflections

On Easter Sunday, the tomb is empty. Angels tell Mary that Jesus is gone. She thinks that something terrible has happened to her Lord. Mary didn't recognize Jesus when he looked like a gardener. Do you recognize me?

On Easter 2009, I prayed to Jesus to be saved. Even though I was symbolically leaving the tomb one year later, I knew that remnants of Maundy Thursday, Good Friday and Easter Saturday were still with me. I know, like in Eliza's story, that I am not invincible. This Easter I could celebrate some aspects of my resurrection, even though I was preoccupied with the cancer possibly returning. I am still learning to live every day to the fullest. I am still learning to let go of my anxieties. I am trying to trust that God has a plan for me and will take care of me, regardless of the outcome. In particular, I know that my level of consciousness for myself, my family, my friends, my work and my spiritual beliefs has expanded.

I never imagined I would write this book. I never imagined I would use a spiritual theme as the dominant paradigm of this or any other written work. But that is what happened. Like a good sociologist, I decided to finish this book by reflecting on my perspective (expanded consciousness), according to the many *roles* I carry. As I listened in church on Easter Sunday, 2010, I decided I wanted to acknowledge the things for which I am grateful. I have begun this reflection with the roles that are external to myself and my family (researcher/educator, sociologist, nurse) and then focused on the more intimate roles (wife, mother, woman, friend, cancer victim, anxious person and, finally, spiritual person).

As a Researcher/Educator

I am grateful I have an advanced education even though I have often had an ambiguous relationship with work. Work could be a major source of stress, but my successes at school and work would often counteract some of my feelings of inferiority that resulted from having a learning disability and general neglect as a child. Five years ago when I was hired as the researcher/educator at the health unit, I thought my ship had really come in. I loved my job and I was very fortunate to have a supportive supervisor, Charlene, and excellent coworkers.

My addiction to the intermittent recognition that I received for my work was a deterrent, however, to finally dealing with the underlying causes of my feelings of inadequacy. It is very clear now that I pushed myself beyond what a reasonable person should do during my illness. For example, instead of following Dr. Potvin's advice to take time off of work while receiving chemo, I asked Charlene if I could work from home. I rationalized I would use sick time when I really needed it. My work did make me feel stronger at times because it was so much a part of my identity; but I also knew I was physically over-taxing myself. At one point when my skin was severely burnt from radiation, I was lying down in bed reading with my notes above my head. It hurt to breathe, but work was such a distraction. I rationalized that as long as I could still think (even though I was not as fast as before chemo), I could not let down my coworkers. My work kept me from thinking about death.

It was not until June 2009 that I began questioning the value of my work. I came into the health unit to make a presentation, even though I still had many physical problems. I shuffled because I could hardly walk from the sciatica. I had absolutely no energy since the fatigue from the radiation and general over-exertion had hit me hard. I physically looked very ill with very dark circles under my eyes and very little hair, which stood up like a mountain peak. My thinking was slow, and I cried easily. It was not surprising the presentation didn't go well. I felt I was to blame and that the organization blamed me. This was the first time I questioned the benefits of work and confirmed for me that I needed to be on part-time disability. I only worked two days per week that summer so I could take more time for healing and become more "capable" of doing my work.

It wasn't until September, when a delayed reaction to my cancer diagnosis and treatment struck and I began having symptoms of post-traumatic stress when I really began to examine the role of work in my recovery. When my family doctor suggested that working full-time might get my mind off of my anxieties, I broke down in tears and went to the cancer clinic counsellor to find out if I was a malingerer (using illness to avoid work). M., my social worker at the cancer clinic, told me to try and listen to my body for a change, so I did. We agreed I would work three days per week until Christmas and use the other two days for recovery, meditation and massage.

It felt like a fatal blow when I found out just before Canadian Thanksgiving that the funding for my job would come to an end May 14th, 2010. I cried, thinking, *Isn't it enough that I have to deal with cancer without having a job loss as well?* I initially recovered, thinking I would have to get better so my family could survive financially. This news forced me to give up my fear of dying as a luxury, and I decided to not worry about a job until the New Year when I was better. I kept hoping that something would happen to save our jobs, but at a meeting held at the end of November, it was very disappointing to discover that the provincial "agency" would not be assuming the research program and staff.

By December, I began questioning whether anyone would want to hire someone as sick as I was. Even though I knew I was sinking into a depression, I decided to go to the nursing curriculum renewal day in December with the university. I was so self-aware of the loss of my "livelihood," just when I really thought that people were valuing my opinion, that I publicly cried about ten times over the two-day period. At that point, I just wanted to be put out to pasture, to never work again. My self-esteem had plummeted.

Just before Christmas, I applied for a temporary job that was posted at the health unit, even though I didn't want to leave the best job of my life until the last moment. I cried when I submitted my resume. I sobbed when human resources called between Christmas and New Year's Day to schedule an interview. The job interview occurred on Epiphany, January 6, 2010. When asked during the interview if I could commit to the job for a year, I started to cry and thought, *I just want to be alive in a year.* When asked what my career plans were in a year, I started to cry again and thought, *I just want to be alive in a year.* Needless to say, I didn't get the job. I was told my answers to the questions were too academic. No one said it was because I was emotionally fragile, but I knew that was also part of the reason for not hiring me.

After my depression was treated in February, I did apply for other positions without even being invited for an interview. I continued to struggle every day as I counted down the days to May 14th, the last day of my job. It became an identity crisis for me. I found it traumatizing to realize I was more psychologically wounded by the loss of my job than the loss of my breasts. I never mourned the loss of my breasts to the same degree that I mourned the loss of my job. I still hope that someone will want to hire me and that my thought processes will be adequate for a job interview. I have some hope about finishing my research and continuing to work as a researcher. I worried about the loss of health and disability benefits, especially given the cost of cancer drugs. I knew that I wasn't the first person to lose my job after experiencing cancer, but cancer and job loss are two major threats to health and well-being.

Andrew, a member of our mediation group, once said to me that we are often addicted to the things that are not healthy for us. I think I have been addicted to work as a way of finding self-worth. My friends tell me I will get a job when I am physically and emotionally ready, and I sincerely want to believe them. I know my *job right now* is to continue to heal, but I continue to barter with God to find a meaningful job, promising that this time I will balance my work and family/personal life. On April 26th, I actually left my house and went for a leisurely lunch with a colleague. It was so affirming. I also saw one of my former professors, and I asked him whether he thought I may be suited for a research position. Not only did he say yes, but he offered to be a reference. Thank you Mary; thank you Bill. I am still trying to convince myself that if I don't get a job right away, I can take a bold step and be off during the summer with my children.

As a Sociologist

I am grateful for being a sociologist because it helped me look at my experience beyond the personal. It is a good thing that society is much more aware of breast cancer compared to twenty years ago. It is staggering to know that one in nine women will get breast cancer in a lifetime. When you think of all of the wives, daughters, friends and coworkers who are affected by this disease, the impact can be phenomenal. The good news is that screening for breast cancer is advancing (although in my case, negative results from the mammogram and ultrasound provided a false security). Breast cancer treatment has also greatly advanced over the past twenty years, and the prognosis for survival is much higher. Is it automatically a death sentence now? No, I don't think so, but I wish I could say all women will be cured. There is still tremendous stress surrounding the uncertainly of whether or not you will be one of the lucky survivors. I do not think there is a negative stigma around breast cancer. Overall we are not blamed for getting our illness, unlike people who are smokers and get lung cancer. I think that breast cancer evokes sympathy and empathy in many people.

I do think the sub-culture of cancer leads to feelings of disempowerment or feelings of being victimized. Because many people with cancer come face to face with death, the cancer sub-culture is an elite club that no one wants to join. Cancer also feels like the master identity that defines you, and all other roles seem to fade, especially when you are so sick you have difficulty fulfilling these other roles, such as worker, mother, wife and friend.[18] You look sick and often act sick. You start to feel self-conscious and think people in the general public are staring at you because you look sick and act sick. Your world becomes more and more insular when you start feeling safe around people who have or had cancer or who treat cancer, thinking they will understand how you are feeling while others not exposed to cancer may not. My fear of having my chemo delayed because of infection was so pronounced that I felt my only choice was to narrow my social milieu. As you get progressively more tired from treatment and its various complications, it becomes easy to be passive and let others tell you what to do and when to do it. The predictability of the treatment routine becomes all-consuming. Personally, I felt like I was an impostor of a functioning person.

When treatment is over, you are introduced to a new social construct: survivor! Now I began understanding that the word *survivor* is a bigger social construct than *victim*. What does it actually mean to be a survivor? Being alive is so much more than just breathing. Can you be a victim and a survivor at the same time? Anthony Giddens, a sociologist, talks of "agency" as referring to the power and choices individuals have relative to their social position.[19] What choices could I really make in my place in the world? I chose to live, but was that choice really under my control? Cancer treatment does not come with guarantees. Sometimes I envy people who talk like they have all of the time in the world to do something or see themselves as having a definite future that they control. I don't have a sense of certainty about anything, beyond knowing that I love my family and friends even when they are occasionally frustrating. Social researchers have discussed the benefits of having an optimistic personality. Do pessimists survive as well?

I also thought of Irving Goffman, a sociologist who studied how people portray themselves to others.[20] What do we hide from others? Do we exaggerate anything? It was very clear that when people asked how we were doing, our family tended to say "good" or "fine," but this wasn't really true. It meant that we were making it through the day or just making it. Sometimes it was an outright lie because it made me feel more vulnerable to know that other people were aware we weren't coping. I was mistrustful. I had too often discovered when I was young that people would kick you when you were down. It was best not to self-disclose weakness. Perhaps I was in denial and didn't want to think about our vulnerability. I gave vague clues, even to my close friends. Sometimes I hid our dysfunction because I didn't want people to worry about us. I just played this game of pretending I was coping because maybe it would become self-prophesy. "How are you?" can be a dreaded question since it becomes a question of whether to lie or not to lie. Maybe it is a good thing that people find out over time you are not coping because you no longer have the energy to maintain an illusion. The secret and shame are out. You become forced to tell others and learn to trust that kindness may come your way.

One of the strangest experiences after being constantly afraid of imminent death is adjusting to the idea of having a future. You try to think about your future until something reminds you of the risk of the cancer returning and you become afraid again. When people ask me what I want in one year, I silently reply to myself, "I would like to be alive." After being a *survivor* for one year, I am beginning to have short periods in the day when I actually forget that I had breast cancer until something happens to reminds me.

As a sociologist, I became amazed about the number of times that breasts and breast cancer come up in general conversation. People make gallows humour like "at least it isn't breast cancer." How is your bra fitting? Sometimes I feel quite surrounded by these conversations and they remind me of the suffering that I experienced. I stay silent when they occur. I don't identify myself as a survivor because I am still mentally unsure that I am a survivor. Perhaps as I survive over time I will become less sensitive or narcissistic when I hear these conversations.

Being a sociologist also helped me analyze whether there are social injustices, such as discrimination. I think people with breast cancer face three types of institutionalized discrimination: 1) drug companies, 2) insurance companies and 3) companies that sell breast prostheses. When I was a university lecturer teaching sociology of the health care system, I would focus on how the drug companies made exorbitant profits on the illness of people because drugs can certainly save lives. Drug companies rationalize exorbitant company profits by suggesting they are covering the costs of developing new drugs. The degree of profit, however, contradicts the illusion that the drug companies are "hard done by." I am grateful I could take the drugs (chemo, the white blood cell stimulant and the estrogen suppressant). I am blatantly aware, however, that we could not have afforded the white blood cell stimulant if my benefit plan at work didn't pay for it. I am very grateful for my pre-existing benefit plan. Knowing that funding for my job ended May 14, 2010, I lament about the thousands of dollars we will pay each year for the estrogen suppressant. I cry for women or anyone with cancer who never had benefits and live in poverty. Do they go without because of their poverty? People in Canada do not generally think you can go bankrupt because of an illness. Outpatient drugs can make you bankrupt in Canada. A national drug plan and access to psychological and registerd massage services could really make a difference to the quality of life of many people with cancer.

There is also discrimination by institutions that sell insurance. You need to have life insurance before you get cancer because you won't get it again. If you are lucky to get if after diagnosis, then you will probably be subjected to the social construct of "pre-existing condition." What exactly does this mean? I think insurance companies are very strategic in disqualifying people. Will insurance companies be able to connect every future illness to my pre-existing condition? Will I never be able to travel again and have travel insurance?

Lastly, I also believe that the cost of prostheses and bras are discriminatory. Other than movie stars, who pays over $80 for a bra? Are the cost of these products so expensive because the Ontario government helps pay? Is there shame associated with a mastectomy so that we cannot wear clothes without breast prostheses? Are we less of a woman if we choose to forgo these prostheses?

Tanya, a woman in my meditation group, mentioned that people who undergo cancer treatment are Olympians, just as much as athletes. There is much work to be done to make the world a more comfortable place for people who experience cancer.

As a Nurse

I am grateful that I am a nurse because this background gave me more information about cancer and the care of someone with cancer than the average person. I knew what questions to ask. On the negative side, I also knew everything that could go wrong and this added to my already high level of anxiety.

Many nurses made a big difference to my life during the period of diagnosis and treatment. Pat and Lynn (nurse practitioners) and Mary-Anne (clinic nurse) were invaluable in going over and over the information when I had questions. They provided excellent advice about how to take care of myself and instilled a sense of hope.

The chemo nurses and triage nurses at the cancer clinic were also superb. They would go over the treatment, ask me about my symptoms and give me advice. I felt very special when a nurse rearranged her assignment so she could give me my last chemo. The nurse during my day surgery who showed me her breast after reconstruction gave me immediate reassurance. She also made me feel like there is life after cancer in which you could look absolutely wonderful. The nurse who listened to my sobbing caused by eight months of built-up fear, anxiety and frustration after that disastrous night in the emergency room was an angel. She bathed me and put me to bed; she rescued me from an abyss. I am sure that she had other tasks that she needed to do while I was sobbing, but she made me feel like I was the only person she was taking care of that morning.

Some nurses left me with a feeling of "wanting." The second night I had to go to the emergency room, I was embarrassed for the nurses who were whining about their personal lives and flirting with the male doctors. I also wish the nurse in the radiation clinic who corrected me about the proper application of the creams to my radiation burn could have done so in a less judgmental and more supportive way. Nurses need to be careful about how they communicate with patients. Yes, I rubbed in the steroid cream because it indirectly helped me scratch the terrible itch of the initial stages of radiation burn. Nurses tend to rub in other creams to get to the deeper layers of skin. It was an innocent mistake, but her comments made me feel like I should have known better. I don't think she knew I felt demeaned; I just think she did not question the impact of her approach on me. I also wish that the nurse who was inexperienced in putting in IVs would not have tried to insert an IV into my last remaining vein. Why can't we admit something is beyond us, rather than being afraid to say we didn't try? Why can't the health care system let people seek help without having to have already tried it first? I can really understand why patients don't complain about the health care system because they feel vulnerable; they may need those particular services in the future and do not want to jeopardize future care.

I truly believe in the theory that many people would prefer to receive services in their home if possible. Hospitals have a lot of germs (hospital acquired infections), and many families are already giving basic care to their families in the hospital because the nurses are overworked with the various functional tasks rather than spending time finding out what is really on the patient's and their family's minds.

If patients have neoadjuvant therapy (chemotherapy for months ahead of surgery), I think that they should be an inpatient at least the first night to make sure there aren't complications. Let the patients ask to go home rather than to ask or "beg" to stay. For the first few days after discharge from the hospital, I think that post-mastectomy patients should be cared for by a registered nurse rather than a registered practical nurse to help prevent complications. Patients need some predictability about home appointments because it helps them feel there is some control in their lives. It can be stressful waiting all day to find out when the nurse is coming to help them. Community nursing services need to be augmented so that the community nurses are not run off their feet trying to work with inadequate resources.

Based on my experience teaching community and family nursing, my main advice is for the nurses to slow down and listen attentively to their patients; maybe the message of suffering is what needs to be heard first. An affirmation of suffering can sometimes lead to a feeling that you are able to continue moving ahead. Having a perfectly changed wound dressing does not mean the patient has the will to live or the energy to cope with day-to-day living. Nurses also really need to ask how the family is doing because I do not think I am alone in feeling that my family was a major drain on my daily levels of energy. The cancer clinic really needs more services to help with the stresses that children face. Even with some of my concerns, overall, I was very grateful for the services of my nurses and the whole treatment team.

Marilyn, a nursing professor I know, called me in February 2010, to ask if I would be willing to talk to the nursing students about my experience and family resiliency. I have not spoken publicly since my diagnosis, since I was fortunate to have someone else present on my behalf. Even at the end of March, I knew I still did not have the energy able to fulfill this request, especially given the intimate and emotional nature of our experience, so I decided to prepare a talk about resilience using a section from the book chapter "Family Nursing" that my colleague Julia and I were submitting [21]. I have included excerpts from this chapter that focus on the message about resiliency, rather than repeat the content of the book.

> Black and Lobo describe **family resilience** as "the successful coping of family members under adversity that enables them to flourish with warmth, support, and cohesion."[22] Family resilience factors can be developed across the life span, yet they are often enhanced during experiences of problem-solving when stressors are subdued. Community Health Nurses (CHNs) must have the conviction to assist the family to identify their strengths, to secure extra-familial resources, and to identify their potential for growth through use of family protective and recovery factors. Family protective and recovery factors may include:
> * Having a positive outlook (optimism, confidence, and humour);
> * Spirituality (belief system of hope and triumph);
> * Family member accord (cohesion, nurturance, avoidance of parental conflict);
> * Flexibility (stable family roles, situational and developmental adjustments);
> * Family communication (clarity, collaborative problem solving);

* Financial management (family warmth despite financial problems); and

* Family time (togetherness with tasks).

I know many people would look at our family and describe us as resilient. The bigger question for me is whether we (as a family) would describe ourselves as resilient. Clearly there were moments when my fears of dying and the side effects of the cancer treatment were "torture." The members of my family are all survivors (my friend Dale uses the word *conquerors*), and there is no doubt we have grown as a family from our experiences. It would be hard for me to talk of resilience during the treatment and recovery. At that time, resilience was primarily a goal I hoped would happen. Hearing people mention that we were resilient during the process only made me feel more like an impostor. I can better articulate my thoughts now after twenty-two months from the beginning of my treatment. I have used Black and Lobo's criteria to describe my beliefs about our family's resilience:

• *Having a positive outlook (optimism, confidence, and humour)*

Every time someone said to me, "You have such a positive outlook," I would cringe inside. Yes, I know the research suggests that people with an optimistic attitude are associated with positive outcomes, but I was not optimistic. I don't think I am the only person who is fearful and anxious. On the optimistic side, though, it is hard for me to believe that all fearful and anxious people are doomed. I think that when we make this type of statement we discourage people from really talking about what is on their minds. It is important to let the family take the lead when seeking feedback. Sometimes affirmations can have a negative effect, and you won't know it unless the family tells you.

- *Family member accord (cohesion, nurturance, avoidance of parental conflict)*

We only have a couple of rules in our house: No hitting; think of other people's feelings; and be co-operative. Kevin and I only focused on a few rules (really values) because we knew we would be unable to implement a long list of rules. Behavioural conditioning in psychology tells you that inconsistent reinforcement is the worst in terms of behavioural change. You consistently act nine times out of ten, but on the tenth time you do nothing and the other person thinks that you forgot. The individual for whom you want to see a change may test you again to see if you are really serious about the change. It becomes a game of nagging and avoidance.

Did we have family member accord? Maybe we did sometimes. Kevin and Eliza had many struggles before finding ways to effectively listen to each other. Kevin and I also had to realign our relationship. I had to quit trying to save my family from suffering and to try and find ways to support them in the changes. Sometimes I just had to accept that they would suffer and I couldn't stop it. I continued to do my best to nurture my family, but I often questioned my effectiveness because I was so exhausted. We had family cohesion most of the time, because we were all in "it" together. Nevertheless, there were many times we had some pleasure and were happy as a family.

- *Flexibility (stable family roles, situational and developmental adjustments)*

Everyone's role changed during my illness. I continue to try to get the girls to pick up after themselves "right away" without being asked, and when I listen to other parents, I think I will be still trying until Eliza and Leonie leave the nest. I keep trying to get the family to understand that I want to have the energy to listen to the girls and Kevin about their day and what is important to them. The more domestic work everyone in the family does, the less I have to do, giving me more time to focus on my own sense of happiness and pleasure.

Telling children about cancer needs to be directed to their level of development and the social context. Leonie, who was nine years old, was traumatized by the diagnosis. I also believe Leonie was more vulnerable because she had latent anxieties of separation that developed when we adopted her from her foster family in Guatemala (even though we did it lovingly). She must have had a terrible fear of separation anxiety that was remembered physically. Leonie was also more vulnerable to fears of death because her friend's mother died of cancer. She knew firsthand that parents can die of cancer. Most of the time Leonie was inconsolable, and she did not get better until she heard from me that Dr. Potvin said I was free from cancer; she could see that I was getting better, albeit very slowly.

As a young teenager, Eliza sublimated her fears into school. It was just too frightening to face my potential death directly. Eliza's story "Invincible" tells of her trauma, but it was written after my treatment ended. Eliza did not share her fears or fully experience the pain until she felt it was "safe" after the completion of my treatment. Sometimes her adolescent angst made her worry that she needed to be redeemed because of her "attitudes or behaviours" during my illness. We were very fortunate Eliza was as mature as she was when I got sick. I think most adolescents are ego-centric or narcissistic at times. Eliza did not punish me for my illness, and she did listen to my feedback. Kevin was clearly the recipient of much of her anger. Eliza does have much insight into anger and fear; however, there are still times when we have "eruptions" of unresolved anger, such as, "I can't even get angry at you like other teens get angry at their parents because you had cancer." Eliza is right. I don't have the fortitude to be "yelled and screamed at." Even though the episodes are very infrequent, I find them very draining. After each episode, I reflect on how much Eliza needs someone she can trust to talk to about her feelings of anger at her mother. I am often amazed she had so much insight at her age. Eliza is wiser than many adults about suffering and coping.

- *Family communication (clarity, collaborative problem solving)*

Going to a family counsellor was a very good decision. Kevin got out of the cave and I had to learn to let go and get into the cave. I was being defensive at times with my family, and I needed to learn to ask for something without having to explain why I needed it. Kevin is now assisting Eliza with her homework. Leonie is being more assertive. We had family discussion before I was sick, but we had a lot more while I was sick. Family communication and support went better after family counselling.

• *Financial management (family warmth despite financial problems)*

Many people also lose a job when experiencing cancer. I am very grateful that I had an understanding employer and employee benefits during this process. During the fall of 2009, we began a concentrated effort to begin paying off our debt (primarily the beautiful sunroom). This meant we needed to start going without. The girls still ask, "Are we poor?" The answer is probably not. Nevertheless, until I get a new job, we will be living off Kevin's salary for the foreseeable future. I hope that someone will want to employ me again. In the meantime, we will have to pay for my very expensive cancer drugs since my employee drug benefits will be ending. This will mean going without something.

• *Family time (togetherness with tasks)*

Our main approach to spending family time together is during meals. Everyone talks about their day. I still help the girls with their homework. I still spend individual time with each of my daughters every day, sometimes many times during the day because they need me or we just "talk" about what is important in life. Sometimes we do tasks together. It takes energy to complete tasks together, and I would rather they take initiative and independently complete their chores. I prefer to spend my time listening and enjoying each other's company.

• *Shared recreation (develop social and cognitive skills, families that play together)*

The 2009 vacation at the cottage was splendid. Everyone knew I was still ill, but we were all very glad of the opportunity to go to the cottage again. Eliza swam in the lake without a life jacket. Leonie swam in the lake with her life jacket. I wear my life jacket symbolically where people can't see it.

- *Routines and rituals (embedded activities that bring the family closer)*

Most of our rituals surround church and secular holidays. We celebrate Advent, Lent and Easter as seasons and not just days. Eliza, Leonie and I clearly enjoy Halloween. We also regularly share holidays with friends and family. I am going to be much more proactive in enjoying my birthday, my anniversary and Mother's Day than I have been in the past.

- *Support network (individual, family, community to share resources)*

My nephew Mike and his family, Michelle, Livvy and Gilly helped me immensely throughout my whole illness. Because they lived in London, Mike came to work on our house in the first few days after chemo. We also had many opportunities to enjoy their company through meals and visits. Two year old Livvy brought laughter into the house on a constant basis. The birth of Gilly brought a sense of new life to our family as well.

My sister Jean came to live in London and I am very grateful. I now see her on a regular basis, and I feel compassion for her life. We also have the opportunity for frequent visits and phone calls. My brother Bob really helped us when our furnace was in trouble in the middle of winter while I was on chemotherapy. Bob and my nephew Mike also installed our new high efficiency furnace. Bob even travelled to London to make a few visits.

My friends were really there for me on a daily and

weekly basis. Karen, Lesley, Kate and Elaine listened to my fears of dying. Many friends came to visit me at our home and stayed away when they were ill. I received many emails of caring and hope. Our friends drove me to radiation. I even met new friends. Something that I never thought would happen. I let some friendships end.

• *Spirituality (belief system of hope and triumph)*

We are going to two churches now. We still follow the Christian liturgical year and try to grow according to the themes of Advent, Epiphany, Lent and Easter. I am much more spiritual than I was. I spend more time in prayer. My meditation has helped me feel closer to God, and this has helped me heal.

I think people rarely experience an illness in isolation from other crises or unresolved memories or grief from the past. For me, my treatment and recovery were oversaturated with feelings of abandonment, unresolved grief for my mother, feelings of inadequacy and lack of self-worth from my childhood. I started healing when I began dealing with these feelings and memories. Being a nurse and having nurses as friends was a marked advantage for me during my treatment and recovery. It meant I always had a skilled listener to turn to, if I chose. I think many nurses, because of time constraints or lack of comfort with the topic, only pay lip service to understanding a patient's view of illness in the context of his or her life. If only nurses had time to really build a trusting relationship with patients so that they could disclose their true anxieties and fears, I think nurses could really help patients heal the wailing of their souls and free up energy for healing. I think the nursing curriculum needs to spend more time focusing on approaches to understand the relationship between spirituality, nursing and healing. Having cancer was a spiritual crisis, and I had difficulty even talking to my friends about these feelings. My spirituality helped me reconcile my past suffering and gave me more energy to cope with my treatment and recovery. In conclusion, I think the most important question a nurse can ask is "Is there something worrying you?" Perhaps it will be a health question, or perhaps the person will share something that is really worrying them and this worrying may be interfering with healing and quality of life.

As a Friend

I am grateful that my friends helped me feel loved and supported during this trial. It felt really great when my friends talked about their lives and their problems and the solutions they were considering. I felt worthwhile when we had conversations beyond my illness and when they were interested in my opinion.

I know my friends were worried that I would die. They listened to my fears of death but rarely acknowledged theirs. I don't know if this was good or bad. In hindsight I think it was a good choice because I didn't need any more pessimism.

My friends wanted to protect me, especially from news that other friends were ill or that acquaintances had died of cancer. I think that sometimes it is harder hearing this news afterwards. It makes you think that you are more vulnerable than you really thought. I know they did it out of love.

When I continued to sink into the depression and my ability to think seemed to be over, my friends really encouraged me to seek treatment for depression. One friend suggested that I "try and stop the negative self-talk." My medication did help reduce my depression. I am now better at reducing the "negative self-talk."

It is really great to have competent friends. My friends who are nurses or counsellors really listened to what I was thinking and feeling. They were living proof confirming all I had thought about the value of social, functional (meals, driving to appointments), spiritual and informational support. My biggest obstacle was deciding what I should disclose, even to my good friends, and whether I should ask for help. Most of the time I would wait for them to offer help. It was easier to accept an offer of help than to specifically ask for something. I did not want to feel like I was dependent or a burden to anyone else. My normal role was to listen and take care. I should have been more honest with my friends and trusted that they would have been there for me, even if I was needy. My fear of being rejected when needy was my default position that needed to be challenged so I could ask for and accept help. My friends helped me heal.

I am grateful my friends helped to edit this book and give me the confidence to move forward towards publishing. They have listened and helped me become more desensitized to my fears of overly exposing ourselves to strangers who may judge our family harshly when they read the book rather than have compassion. I am very grateful for the gift of making new friends. I rarely made new friends over the past fifteen years because I was so busy with my studies and then my family. I always felt I didn't have time for my old friends, let alone have time to develop new friendships. I am grateful for my new friends because they have also expanded my world view. I am still sad over the lost friendships, just not as sad as I was.

Leonie has also made a new and very strong friendship. One day, she was having a bad morning and was crying, wanting to stay home from school, but I decided she needed to go to school. Casey came on her bike so they could ride to school together. Leonie was still crying when she left the house. Halfway to school, Casey stopped her bike and asked Leonie what was wrong and Leonie told her. Casey said, "Leonie what you need is to be around a good friend all day and have pizza lunch." We all need the wisdom of ten year olds. We all need friends like Casey; friends are invaluable.

As a Wife

I am grateful that Kevin is my husband. When I was first diagnosed, I really didn't give much thought to my role as Kevin's wife beyond finding fault with him. I understand the irony of the last statement and know that my ability to give in our relationship was very limited. Even though I was often frustrated, angry and resentful, I still desired a closer relationship with Kevin. I am very grateful that our marriage survived this period. I know that many marriages fail when cancer strikes.

My fears and neediness dominated our marriage during my cancer treatment. I was very resentful that Kevin could not rise to the occasion, even though he was trying his best. I knew he had to leave for Victoria for work shortly after my diagnosis, and even though I agreed to the trip, I felt deserted having to support the girls while I was falling apart. After that point, though, Kevin came to every one of my subsequent doctor's appointments and gave me emotional support for which I am very grateful. He also took notes so that we could go over what had happened after the appointments.

In November 2008, I told Kevin's counsellor at the cancer clinic how frustrated I was with him when he would say that he would do things and then not follow through. I also felt tremendous frustration when I would ask for something, but he would do what he thought was needed. When I got angry, Kevin would break down and then I would comfort him. We had cycled through this pattern many times during our marriage. During this counselling session, Kevin admitted that he needed to feel uncomfortable to change. I realized I had been setting the scene for perpetual failure by comforting Kevin after I was angry. I discovered I was the one who needed to change. I had to learn to let Kevin feel uncomfortable after a disagreement. As I made progress, he did start to change and do the things he said he was going to do. I felt very grateful when it seemed that he started to listen to what I wanted. He began to understand that during the periods when I was irrational (these things can happen to anyone, but it is far worse on chemo), I would appreciate his support and we could talk about the issue later. This approach really worked and I started to learn to calm down quicker.

Another area of contention was the squabbling between Kevin and Eliza. It was like having two adolescents in the house. I felt very grateful when Kevin began to work on his relationship with Eliza. Even though their problems continued over the next nine months, the squabbles became less extreme. Kevin didn't make a lot of progress with the relationship until we entered family therapy the summer following the end of my radiation treatment. Our counsellor, Pirie, told me to go to "the back of the cave" and for Kevin to "get out of the back of the cave." Pirie began to be a role model for Kevin as the archetypical "good father." The family relationships really started improving after we started family counselling. Even though I was still exhausted and unwell, we were able to go to the cottage and have an enjoyable time.

Starting dancing lessons again that fall was a great *step* forward to bringing joy back into our lives. We were actually touching each other. We were laughing together. We made many mistakes dancing, and it felt like we didn't have a care in the world. We were having fun and being disruptive in class. As time went on, we were actually doing better dancing than before I was sick. We began to be "in synch."

As my neediness decreased, I started to notice and appreciate the things that Kevin was doing. We were becoming more of a team in guiding and supporting the girls, especially Eliza. He moved beyond being a functional helper to really trying to understand how I felt and give me the support that I thought I needed, rather than what he thought I needed. I used to ask what he was going to do, hoping he could give me the answer that I wanted. I now tell him directly when I want him to do something for me. He is better able to set priorities between work and home when I am direct. He really does want to put family first, and gentle reminders help him choose. Kevin decided that he would like just the two of us to go to an inn overnight for his birthday May 2, 2010. We hadn't been away together for about five years. The trip was perfect, a nice dinner, a little romance, more than one nap, all resulting in a deep sense of connectedness. I can honestly say that our marriage is better now than before I was sick. Kevin is not a jerk.

As a Mother

I am grateful for my daughters, Eliza and Leonie. My memories of having a mother are very scant. I just always knew that I wanted my children to not have to experience the pain and neglect of my childhood. I spent a great deal of time with both Eliza and Leonie before I was sick to find out what they were thinking and feeling. I would try to emotionally support them and provide guidance. Sometimes I had to tell them when they were really wrong and not thinking of others. Sometimes this was an exhausting process.

Upon finding out that I had cancer, I really had to deal with my fear of history repeating itself. Every day I was consumed with the fear that I would die and my daughters wouldn't have a mother. I would think, *At least they wouldn't be orphans,* but this was not a comforting thought.

During the stages of early testing and then my treatment, it was clear to me I did not have energy for myself nor my girls, yet my girls were in a crisis! I wish I could have found a better balance with respect to taking care of myself and my girls. My reality was that I did put my girls first, even when I worried it would over tire me and interfere with healing. Sometimes I felt a terrible anger inside thinking that dealing with cancer was enough, without having a family in crisis. It was a good decision to begin "office hours" similar to the set times I would have for my students. Eliza and Leonie both had a set time to bring me their worries and concerns. This process helped during the day, because they would both wait until office hours to tell me what was on their minds. It didn't work in the evening though. Almost every night, I would fall asleep while they were talking. I would often feel so exhausted and think

251

there was no hope for me. It wasn't until after the treatment was over that it was very clear to me that I wouldn't heal until my family started to heal. One of the best decisions I made was to let go of the anger, accept that they did the best they could and forgive them.

I am very glad Lesley suggested family counselling. Pirie could say things that I had said 1,000 times, yet Kevin and the girls actually heard him and started making some changes. I talked about the need for the girls to be able to comfort themselves or for them to go to their father. Pirie told me I did not have to defend my desires to my children. I had always given my girls an explanation for the things that I wanted from them, so they would learn why. I knew Eliza and Leonie already knew the family values, but I would continue to explain why I wanted something. I could see that I was coming across as defensive. I started learning to try and not to defend my position when making a request. I started asking the girls to go to their father for comfort. I would even ask them to leave me when I was really tired and actually mean it. I am still very sensitive to Eliza's and Leonie's feelings of anger and sadness, and I wish I could save them from these harder feelings. We still continue to process the feelings of anger and resentment that originated during my diagnosis and treatment. I know I can't save them from suffering. I am much clearer in knowing I have taught them problem-solving and conflict-resolution skills and that I need to have faith they can practice these skills independently in order to become more confident. If I didn't have the faith they would eventually be able to cope, I would be making them dependent.

At this point, my only complaint (probably like millions of parents everywhere) is that they need to pick up after themselves to reduce the domestic load. I am even making some very slow progress in this area as well. It is very clear to me a person needs to have energy to initiate a change. I needed energy to change, but so did Kevin, Eliza and Leonie. I am currently teaching Eliza and Leonie how to take care of "me." If the girls have done something that has frustrated me and I want them to fix "it," I have started asking them to do my request right away, because it will make me happy. I started using this approach so the girls can relate the impact of their actions to my energy levels and my feelings. I now know I need to role model better treatment towards me, so they in turn will not become self-sacrificing mothers.

Eliza, Leonie and Kevin were my main motivators to fight to live, even though at the time of treatment and recovery, I thought I would literally kill them or they would end up killing me. They are still my motivators, I just don't have the urge to kill them now. They can irritate me, but I don't think they are killing me.

As a Woman

I have always joked with Kevin and my friends that I am more male in my outlook than female. I would tease Kevin that I had more testosterone than him and he had more estrogen than me. After eight months of taking an estrogen suppressant, the latter is probably true.

I don't think I was as traumatized by losing my breasts as some women describe, probably because I have never really felt physically attractive in my life nor very feminine. As I gained weight, my breasts became heavier and they pulled on my neck and shoulders. At age fifty, gravity ensured they were well on their way to sinking down to my waist and no one could ever imagine they were aesthetically pleasing. Their touch, however, was sexually pleasing. The tiredness of cancer and its treatment made me asexual. I do remember wearing a turtleneck sweater the first time we made love; I didn't want to be reminded that my breasts were gone.

I was originally going to get two perky saline implants. I knew I was not willing to have abdominal surgery for implants even if it could reduce my waistline. The complications from surgery were a major deterrent to thinking about breast reconstruction. I am not even sure if it would work because of the significant internal scarring that I had after the radiation burn. Luckily the Ontario government does not have a timeline on when breast reconstruction can occur.

I am adamant that I do not want to wear a bra anymore. If this has happened to me, at least I can be liberated from having to wear a bra. No one can really tell that I do not have breasts during winter because my chest is covered with heavy sweaters or my coat. As spring arrived in 2010, I was beginning to lose some of my self-consciousness about just wearing a light shirt around friends. I am contemplating never wearing a prosthesis or bra again. Maybe if I am comfortable with my "deformity," other people will learn to be comfortable seeing a woman without breasts. I discovered that it is hard for people to look at my chest if I am looking them "straight in the eye," hopefully with a smile.

The cancer treatment took its biggest toll on my facial self-image. I felt self-conscious because at Halloween I looked like Uncle Fester from the Addams Family as my face took on a greyish colour when the steroids thinned my skin and I had such big black circles around my eyes. I did not want to look like Uncle Fester! I thought I looked ugly (and I wasn't even sure what ugly meant). The dark circles under my eyes made me anxious, because I often thought they meant that cancer was lurking, doing undetected damage. For someone who never wore any make-up, I went to a "Look Good, Feel Better" session at the cancer clinic, but I didn't participate in applying make-up. It was not until the antidepressants brought me sleep that the dark circles decreased around my eyes and my skin started to thicken as the effect of the steroid receded. Then I started to think I looked a bit better. The night of the Valentine's Day dance 2010, someone who I hadn't seen since before my cancer told me she wouldn't have known I had cancer if I hadn't told her. I was wearing a beautiful pink and teal cardigan that I had knit almost twenty years before. I did look much better. Thank you to everyone who lied about my appearance. I know you were being sincere when you said I looked good. It was because you had seen me when I looked really, really bad. I recently had my hair curled, and I have started to draw on my eyebrows with an eyebrow pencil because I really do look better. Maybe "Look Good, Feel Better" did have an important message.

It is probably an urban myth that tribal Amazon women would sever a breast as an initiation to becoming a warrior. The breast was considered a hindrance in the use of the bow, and their prowess with the bow could continually improve after this ritual. If this is the case, my double mastectomy may be my first step towards being a warrior.

As a Cancer Victim

I still cannot write the words "I am grateful for having cancer." I know that many good things have happened as well as the bad things. I just can't say the words.

I always fought against seeing myself as a victim just because I was an orphan. I have had many, many major losses over my life and was able to continue to fight, so I didn't initially think of myself as a victim. Eventually the cancer broke me enough so I did start thinking of myself as a victim. The feelings of being a victim did not start right away. I was too shocked to feel a victim even though I did continue to ask the question "Why me?" I really thought that I had experienced more than my share of losses.

The feelings of being a victim often depended upon the situation. I remember thinking I was completely powerless during chemo, so I just stuck out my arm very submissively. The only thing that I could do in the early days of treatment was pray. Like with my miscarriages, I felt there was nothing I could do to change the inevitable. I did think that my prayers for others would be heard though. Thus, I decided that my major activity during the rough days of chemo would be to pray for others. Kate comforted me when she said, "What makes you think prayer is not work?"

When I think about the time period when I was having chemo, I did not feel like a complete victim because I believed the chemo was saving my life. I could take action by exercising and eating well. In addition, by choosing to take the drug that stimulated my white blood cells to increase my resistance to infection allowed me to have guests over to visit, thus reducing my feelings of isolation and being a victim.

In contrast, the feelings of being a victim really began when I started having trouble making decisions (chemo brain). I had anticipated that chemo would be the hardest portion of my treatment, so when I survived the chemo, I really thought I would get back on my feet quickly. Even though I was terribly afraid of dying during the surgery, I managed to sit up after the surgery and walk to the bathroom; after arriving home after the day surgery, I independently walked up the stairs to my bedroom with a surgical drain in each hands. Perhaps the process of feeling victimized occurred because I did not worry about post-surgical complications, and I was really wrong. It was the complications that really convinced me I was a victim. I knew that hemorrhage could kill because in the past I was an intensive care nurse. The night I bled, I wondered if I should stay still to make sure the bleeding did not get worse. I felt powerless when Jodi took me to emergency and I was convinced that people in the emergency room were staring at me, confirming that I looked terrible and very ill. When I came home, I was still feeling like a victim. The night I woke up with blood all over when the drain came apart, I cried out to Jodi and she came. I felt like a baby being washed and having my sheets changed in the middle of the night. I felt at the mercy of home care, not knowing when they would come to visit. I let them make the decisions about things I would have normally decided myself, such as when to call the doctor.

The day I became chilled from the initial signs of sepsis, I could ask Kevin to take me to the emergency room and I felt cared for the first night at emergency. Even the next day when the chills returned, I was able to call Dr. Holiday and when he asked whether I thought that I should return to the hospital, I could assert myself and say "Yes." It was the second night I went to the emergency room that I completely "broke" and felt like I was a "total victim." I thought I would die from the sepsis and no one would notice nor care. That night when I returned to the emergency room, I could not assert myself and felt very vulnerable. I felt even more vulnerable when I stood up to go to the bathroom and all of this old blood came pouring out my right drain site. Kevin, who I felt was my only advocate that night, had to leave at 10:30 p.m. to go home to the girls, and all I could do was listen to the idle chatter of disinterested staff. Even though I had been a director of nursing for many years, I never complained. I stayed silent. I stayed silent or hysterical while worrying; I was passive. I tried unsuccessfully to assert myself in interacting with the community nurse. By now, I had totally integrated the role of victim. Come here, go there, I just did as I was told.

I stayed very passive during most of my experience of Easter Saturday. The feelings of passivity and powerlessness accumulated during my depression. I did choose to get treatment for the depression only because I felt desperate with suicidal thoughts. The antidepressants awoke me from my overall feelings of being a victim. I am still amazed that it only took two weeks on the proper drug for some of my self-confidence to begin to return and my thinking to be clearer (just not at my pre-chemo level). Now I am awakening like the spring after a long winter. I have no desire to fight with anyone. If I think that something needs to be done, but I do not have the energy to do it myself, I ask someone who I think is capable to do it and I wait.

Right now as I passed the one-year milestone after my last dose of radiation, I am beginning to feel like a survivor. I feel more like I am a victim of job loss rather than cancer. I passed my last visit to Dr. Potvin and Dr. Powers on June 2, 2010, and I do not need another follow-up visit for six months. Joanne, my massage therapist, told me I could start stretching in readiness to swing a golf club. It is much harder to believe that I am a victim when I am going to be able to play golf. (Others may say there is nothing like a golf course to help you feel like you are a victim.) I guess there are degrees of victimization and "once a victim, does not mean always a victim."

As an Anxious Person and a Daughter

I am going to learn to be grateful that I am an anxious person. Maybe this exercise will finally convince me I am worthy. My anxiety of an early death was a very negative approach to remembering my mother and my grandfather. I longed to be a daughter, but I knew it could never happen. I now know a lot more about mothering because I have been a mother to my daughters. I can see how mothers can comfort and nurture daughters and build their self-confidence.

In the spring of 2010, I started to meditate on what it would be like to be with my mother and I would tell her the things I would like her to know. I asked my older sisters and brother if they had a picture of my mother, because up until then I did not have one. I believed a picture might make her feel more real to me. Now I try to spend some time remembering my mother and grandfather directly, instead of indirectly through fear. Maybe if I had had a mother when I was young, I would not have been so anxious most of my life because she could have affirmed and reassured me. Sometimes I imagine what it would have been like to have a mother during my cancer treatment. She may have taken care of me and my family. She may have made some meals, done laundry, listened to all of our fears (especially mine) and kissed us all better.

Just like in the Charles Dickens novel *A Christmas Carol*, I know that I had a "bah humbug" attitude towards Mother's Day my whole life. This year Kevin and I went out to buy a tree to commemorate both my mother and me. I chose a "twisted lavender weeping rosebud." We had a barbeque on Mother's Day, and I invited my whole family. It is ironic and very symbolic that I started my journey with cancer with a family barbeque on Labour Day and now I am ending this part of the journey with a family barbeque on Mother's Day. Before dinner, I took out the picture of my mother and held it up. I started to sob when I showed the picture to Eliza and Leonie. I continued to sob when I asked everyone in the room to remember or think kindly of our mother. It was very cathartic to admit my grief to my family when I clearly realized that I have denied my grief for almost fifty years. Like Scrooge on Christmas morning, I will always keep the spirit of Mother's Day in my heart and soul 365 days of the year.

My anxieties also taught me to be a strategic person and develop contingency plans to keep me safe. Even though many of my fears did not come true, I had a plan in case they did. I really realize my anxieties are from the same gene that gave me my creativity. The gene that enables me to experience "virtual reality" in exploring new ways of viewing phenomena is also the gene that stimulates catastrophic thinking. In reality, I do not think I would give up my creativity in exchange for losing the anxiety.

Is my anxiety a physical condition? Absolutely! Am I hypochondriac? No, I am not; hypochondriacs really believe they have the illness. Instead I was ashamed of my preoccupation with my health and constant fears of dying. Is my anxiety a mental illness? If it is, it is probably one of the oldest illnesses going. Everyone gets anxious. Yes, I am anxious, but more often than not I can still be high functioning. My cancer was my crossroads. I could not longer "hide" my anxieties. My illness, however, was being ashamed of being anxious. I want to live to be a ripe old age and hopefully enjoy grandchildren. Because I am a nurse, I will probably notice any physical anomalies, wonder if the things that I notice are serious and continue to be overwhelmed. I am learning to be more patient and less anxious while I wait to find out if my fear is actually true. My pimple or skin problem has now healed even though I panicked, worrying that the cancer had returned. I just have to try and be patient without jumping to conclusions or be kind to myself when I am jumping to conclusions. I am going to others for advice and support so that I do not carry my worry alone.

I am also trying to learn to be a more grounded person and take care of myself. Following Helen's advice, I am learning self-care by watching our cat. Cats know how to get love from people and intrinsically know how to take care of themselves. I am very glad my friends and health care providers accepted my anxiety without judgment, or at least as far as I know they did. Being anxious doesn't need to be the master identity. Maybe people will see my master identity as a very caring, sensitive and creative person. If I am gentle with myself, I may even have more energy for healing.

As a Spiritual Person

I am grateful that I am a spiritual person. When I was a little girl, I often thought God was the only one who cared about me. I thought I had a guardian angel to travel with me and protect me, because no one else would. I still carry these beliefs.

I am very familiar with being angry at God because I have experienced far too many losses to not wonder if I was a bad person and if it was deserved. Does God really only give you what you can handle? I don't always think so because I have been in over my head way too many times.

Cancer can be a spiritual crisis because you come face to face with death. Will God shrink my tumour? What am I supposed to learn? Am I learning?

> I have learned to let go of most of my pain and resentment as a child.
> I have learned to let go of the pain and resentment of multiple miscarriages.
> I can no longer take on the pains and injustices of the world.
> I can pray for people experiencing suffering and injustice in the world.
> Physical, emotional and spiritual healing can occur in the midst of chaos.
> Frequent communion helped me to feel like I could heal.

In the past, I never gave much thought to Jesus. When I was younger, I could never get past the fact that he was male. As I got older, I was alienated by all of the patriarchy. Instead, I primarily thought of God, and my images of God were nurturing and female. It is completely surprising to me still that I have written this entire book using the passion of Jesus as the central theme. I have never thought so much about Jesus in my whole life. After my experience with cancer, it is easier to think of Jesus as androgynous. I am getting more comfortable thinking about what his life was like and the messages he was sent to bring to a suffering people.

I think people with cancer need the opportunity to explore spiritual questions and beliefs with someone in pastoral care and or someone who can listen because he or she has already found meaning in suffering. I used a Christian perspective to frame my journey. Another Christian could have a completely different perspective. Someone from a different religion or spiritual grounding would also have different perspectives. I think what is important is that they have an opportunity to voice their thoughts and beliefs during the process of healing to bring restoration, healing and acceptance.

For me, I would think about the scripture reading every week for a message of guidance or comfort. Weekly communion was healing and gave me fortitude. Kate's laying on of healing hands helped me; disclosing my shame on Good Friday was freeing. My silent spiritual retreat to Medaille House reaped many benefits. I walked the labyrinth to seek understanding of what is sacred in my life. An example of this would be remembering my mother and telling her what I would like her to know. I also experienced solitude and peace in isolation away from my family; even all of my meals were made for me. Kate, Sister C., Mona and Helen have had tremendous influence on my recovery and spiritual beliefs. One of the things I have promised myself in the future is to schedule regular spiritual retreats. I think that by taking care better care of myself, I may have more energy for my family, friends and work.

My meditation group has been the most healing experience of my life. I have thoroughly enjoyed the fellowship of the group. I think and pray for the group, members present and the members who can't come to particular sessions. Regardless of their physical presence, we are together. I think meditation has brought calmness to my soul. I begin my meditation silently reciting the Lord's Prayer and the Lord is My Shepherd. I have connected with a place in my soul that has allowed me to heal past wounds as well as my wounded body from cancer. Mediation opened a window for conversation between my conscious and subconscious with God. It has been a time of healing and hope. The metta (the Buddhist meditation of loving kindness) has promoted loving kindness in my soul towards others. I can easily forgive others and ask forgiveness. I have no desire to be angry at anyone, even those promoting injustice. I told Deborah, our leader, that I am the one to coin metta as a verb rather than a noun. If I am upset, I just start saying metta for that person because it is impossible to say metta and be angry at the same time. I still carry many frustrations, but I am using metta to make my way through them. Deborah says the Buddha taught his followers metta as an antidote for fear. I am still afraid but not as much. Meditation has been a "sacred" time for me.

I know I had two cancers, a physical one (breast cancer) and an emotional one (pessimism, fear, anxiety, blame and doubt). I am not usually maudlin, but as my breasts were severed off, this surgical act brought my heart closer to the surface. I have begun to understand spirituality at a much deeper level, which most likely wouldn't have happened without this cancer. I really realize my biggest "sin" has been the lack of faith or trust in God to take care of me. (Kate tells me this is not a sin though.) I have often been on the periphery of this trust but could never internalize it over time. People talk about cancer as being life transforming, and I know I am no longer the person I was before the cancer struck. I am not even the person I was a year ago as I began my recovery. I have to cope with daily frustrations by being more assertive and trying to appreciate the moment, focusing on what is good rather than what has not been completed. I am still learning to live and be grateful in the moment and find joy in my day-to-day existence. I am more open to these ideas now.

I am ending this book with my sermon that I presented at the end of the Easter season. I prepared my sermon weeks in advance. I was a little nervous before I started, but shortly after I started, I put away my notes and let God help me. We all cried a little.

Hosannas
May 16, 2010

Probably for the past five years I have wanted to give a sermon. I don't know why. I typically shy away from public speaking unless it is through my work. I am here today because I asked Mona if I could speak one Sunday. Mona, being the affable person that she is, said, "Yes." I chose this Sunday, the seventh Sunday in Easter, because it is especially important to me in my recovery from advanced breast cancer.

First, I would like to seriously thank everyone for your support of our family during the past twenty months. Kevin and I came to Hosannas August 31, 2008. I had just been diagnosed with the locally advanced breast cancer. I was feeling tired and hopeless. Kevin and I knew Kate and Alistair (mainly Alistair) for a long time, and I had a feeling I would be safe here at Hosannas. I felt welcome even though I was afraid to shake hands during the sign of peace. You have all adapted to shaking my left hand, but you may not know it is because I am afraid that shaking my right arm may damage it again. You have welcomed us and made us honorary Anglicans just by showing up for three months. I was safe. I am safe. We are safe. We thank you.

There are a couple of themes from today's readings that I want to emphasize. In the Psalm, I think the main message is that God is powerful and protects us. John 17 verse 26 says, "I have made you known to them, and will continue to make you known in order that the love you have for me may be in them and that I myself may be in them" (NIV). We need to feel "one" with God. In Revelation 22:17 we hear, "Whoever is thirsty, let him come; and whoever wishes, let him take the free gift of the water of life" (NIV).

In the reading from Acts, I see the patriarchal world of Paul. No one is rebelling because the slave woman is a slave. No one is rebelling when her fortune telling is true. She is like the town crier (like Paul Revere: "the British are coming!").

Paul and Silas *are* servants of the Most High God and are telling people the way to be saved.

In the Good News Bible we are told that Paul is upset with this behaviour. In the New International Version, Paul is troubled. Neither version tells us why. I would like to believe that it is because she is being used to make money for the slave owners. Her fortune telling is true but *not* free.

In true Marxist style, the slave owners are angry that their source of profits are dried up when Paul exorcizes the spirit. The Roman citizens become a mob and stripped and beat Paul and Silas. Paul and Silas are thrown into jail. It appears that taking away someone's (i.e. the slave owners) living is against the law in ancient Rome.

I don't know about you, but I probably don't have the resiliency to be stripped, beaten, thrown in jail, put in stocks and still be able to sing hymns. I can truly understand how Paul and Silas would want to pray. We don't know what they were praying for though.

Just like on Good Friday at 3:00, when an earthquake happens and tears the curtain of the temple, we hear again that an earthquake breaks away the prison door to enable Paul and Silas to go free. In Roman times, failure to do your job may mean death. The jailer decides to take his life before the public humiliation of having his prisoners escape. Paul saves the jailor from taking his life by crying out that they are still there. The jailer has not failed in his job. The jailer sees that a miracle has happened, through Paul's God, and wants to be saved. In gratitude, the jailer takes Paul and Silas to his home and cares for them. The jailer believes in God/Jesus and is joyful that he is saved.

What does this passage mean to us today? I think that many people have experienced injustices in life and have literally been beaten and thrown in jail. I also think that some people end up in a figurative jail because of a trauma, like my cancer, which was not deserved.

I have been giving the Easter season a great deal of thought. I have written a book about our family's experience of locally advanced breast cancer. Last year I prayed at Easter to be saved and I am cancer free, even though I still worry that it will come back. During my recovery I have learned to meditate. I often think that is the time in which I am "one" with God. During one of my meditations, I got the feeling I should write my book according to the Easter passion paradigm. I worried before my diagnosis and the early diagnostic tests and tried to relate it to Jesus' experiences in the wilderness and Gethsemane. I tried to relate to Jesus' suffering on the cross during the many complications from chemo, a double mastectomy and radiation. I think that my biggest epiphany was finally learning to understand that we need to take time on Easter Saturday to retreat to the tomb. We need to retreat to find meaning in suffering and healing before the release on Easter Sunday. I feel the redemption of Easter. I also think that resurrection is about learning to trust again even though something bad has happened—that God will take care of us. God was with us during our suffering, and God will be with us in good times and bad. God can take away any anger and shame. We can be forgiven.

I don't think I had this kind of faith in the past. I experienced tragedy early in life, and I think I have always lived my life anxious about when the next "shoe would be dropped." I could easily pray for others, but I had a difficult time praying for myself. My challenge is to have faith that God will take care of me, because She has taken care of me in the past during times of little trouble and big trouble. I have decided to reword one line in the 23rd Psalm. Instead of having a table prepared in the presence of my enemies, I prefer that God prepare a table for me, my loved ones, and my enemies. Maybe a good meal will help us forget what we were upset or worried about. Maybe I have been my own worst enemy. I have also begun to wonder if God has time to take care of Herself. Like many mothers, maybe God constantly has to take care of others and fix things? I sometimes pray that God finds time to rest to take care of Herself and find time for pleasure and beauty in her creation.

Jesus taught in parables to help people explore the meaning of important things. I am going to end this sermon with my parable.

> There once was a woman who lost her way.
> Fear and death were shadows creeping up trying to overcome her.
> Then one Good Friday, chemo took her hair; the scalpel took her breast; radiation burned her flesh; lack of faith sapped her dignity.
> For forty days and forty nights, she was nestled in the tomb of Easter Saturday.
> The light of Easter Sunday beckoned her forth to repeat the message of Revelation: "Whoever is thirsty, let him come; and whoever wishes, let him take the free gift of the water of life."

We don't have to pay slave owners for this message. It is free. I think the water of life is feeling that we are one with God. The Easter message is to sing unto the Lord and rejoice in the strength of our salvation. We need to come before Her presence with thanksgiving and show ourselves glad in Her with psalms.[23]

After May 22, 2010, we end the season of Easter and will enter the season of Pentecost. Mona describes Pentecost as the season of "regular" Christian living. I will be headed back to the normal world where I will try to continue to make a difference. I hope our book will help people to pray and dance with God should they experience a spiritual crisis as a result of a disease or some other type of traumatic loss. I think there is certain "sacredness" to our book. We have poured out our suffering and struggle to heal. We are trying to find pleasure and sacredness in daily living. We have given "acts" of kindness and received acts of kindness in return. I have been told to "take up my bed and walk." Maybe good things can happen to us with God as our keeper. The grace of God is among us (Revelation 22:21).

Endnotes

[1] A pseudonym

[2] We nicknamed the girls' godmother Mary Poppins about ten years ago.

[3] "Eat this Bread, Drink this Cup. Hymn #63," in *Common Praise Anglican Church of Canada*. (Toronto, ON: Anglican Book Centre, 1998).

[4] Bernie Siegel, *Love, Medicine and Miracles: Lessons Learned about Self-Healing from a Surgeon's Experience with Exceptional Patients*. (Minneapolis, MN: Quill Publishing, 1986).

[5] Pema Chrödrön, *The Places that Scare You: a Guide to Fearlessness in Difficult Times*. (Boston, MA.: Shambhala, 2001).

[6] James Wilkes, *The Gift of Courage*. (Toronto, ON: Anglican Book Centre, 1979).

[7] David Giuliano, *Postcards from the Valley: Encounters with Fear, Faith and God*. (Toronto, ON: United Church Publishing House, 2008).

8 "On Eagle's Wings," in *Voices United: The Hymn and Worship Book of the United Church of Canada* (Etobicoke, ON: The United Church Publishing House, 1996. 808).

9 "La ténèbre n'est point ténèbre. Hymn #549," in *Common Praise Anglican Church of Canada* (Toronto, ON: Anglican Book Centre, 1998).

10 "I Danced in the Morning. Hymn #352," in *Voices United: The Hymn and Worship Book of the United Church of Canada* (Etobicoke , ON: The United Church Publishing House, 1996).

11 Sue Monk Kidd. *Dance of the Dissonant Daughter: A Woman's Journey from Christian Tradition to the Sacred Feminine*. (New York, NY: Harper/Collins, 1996).

12 Sherri Magee and Kathy Scalzo, *Picking up the Pieces: Moving Forward After a Cancer Diagnosis*. (Vancouver, BC: Raincoast Books, 2006).

13 Abraham Maslow. *Religion, Values and Peak Experiences*. (New York, NY: Viking, 1970).

14 Henry Nouwen, *Can You Drink the Cup?* (Tenth Anniversary Edition). (Notre Dame, IN: Ave Maria Press, 2006.)

15 Marion Woodman, *Bone: A Journal of Wisdom, Strength and Healing*. (Toronto ON: Penguin Compass, 2001.)

16 Carl Jung, *Memories, Dreams, Reflections*. (New York, NY: Pantheon Books, 1963.)

17 I had a follow-up appointment with Dr. Holiday, my surgeon, and Pat, his nurse practitioner on April 6, 2010. They examined my "pimple." Neither of them made me

feel foolish to be worried about a pimple. Both thought the pimple was not a return of the cancer. Dr. Holiday was going to excise it on April 28, 2010, so that I could have "peace of mind," but to my surprise it did heal after ten weeks. My health care team has been invaluable in helping me not only deal with the physical illness, but also my fear and anxiety.

[18] Bruce Links, et al. "Socio-Economic Status and Schizophrenia: A Modified Labeling Theory Approach to Mental Disorders: An Empirical Assessment," *American Sociological Review* 54 (1989):400-423.

[19] Anthony Giddens. *The Constitution of Society: Outline of the Theory of Structuration.* (Berkeley, CA: University of California Press, 1984).

[20] Erving Goffman. *The Presentation of Self in Everyday Life.* (Garden City, NY: Doubleday Anchor Books, 1959.)

[21] Patricia Sealy and Julia Smith *"Family Nursing" in Community Nursing 3rd Edition. ed.* Lynette Stamler and Lucia Yu. (Toronto: Pearson, 2011).

[22] Keri Black and Marie Lobo. "A Conceptual Review of Family Resilience Factors," Journal of Family Nursing 14(1) (2008): 38.

[23] Venite, Exultemus Domino. *The Book of Common Prayer and Administration of the Sacraments and Other Right and Ceremonies of the Church According to the Use of the Anglican Church of Canada.* (Cambridge, England: Cambridge University, 1959.)

References

Chrödrön, Pema. *The Places that Scare You: a Guide to Fearlessness in Difficult Times*. Boston, MA.: Shambhala, 2001.

Common Praise: Anglican Church of Canada. Toronto, ON: Anglican Book Centre, 1998.

Black, Keri and Marie Lobo. "A Conceptual Review of Family Resilience Factors, Journal of Family Nursing,14(1) (2008): 33-55.

Giddens, Anthony. *The Constitution of Society: Outline of the Theory of Structuration*. Berkeley, CA: University of California Press, 1984.

Giuliano, David. *Postcards from the Valley: Encounters with Fear, Faith and God*. Toronto, ON: United Church Publishing House, 2008.

Goffman, Erving. *The Presentation of Self in Everyday Life*. Garden City, NY: Doubleday Anchor Books, 1959.

Jung, Carl. *Memories, Dreams, Reflections*. New York: Pantheon Books, 1963.

Kidd, Sue Monk. *Dance of the Dissonant Daughter: A Woman's Journey from Christian Tradition to the Sacred Feminine*. New York, NY: Harper/Collins, 1996.

Links, Bruce et al. "Socio-Economic Status and Schizophrenia: A Modified Labeling Theory Approach to Mental Disorders: An Empirical Assessment," *American Sociological Review* 54 (1989):400-423.

Magee, Sherri and Kathy Scalzo. *Picking up the Pieces: Moving Forward After a Cancer Diagnosis*. Vancouver, BC: Raincoast Books, 2006.

Maslow, Abraham. *Religion, Values and Peak Experiences*. New York, NY: Viking, 1970.

Nouwen, Henry J.M. *Can you drink the cup?* (Tenth Anniversary Edition). Notre Dame, IN: Ave Maria Press, 2006.

Siegel, Bernie. *Love, Medicine and Miracles: Lessons Learned about Self-Healing from a Surgeon's Experience with Exceptional Patients*. Minneapolis, MN: Quill Publishing, 1986.

Sealy, Patricia and Julia Smith *"Family Nursing" in Community Nursing 3rd Edition. ed.* Lynette Stamler and Lucia Yu. Toronto: Pearson, 2011.

Venite, Exultemus Domino (Psalm 95). *The Book of Common Prayer and Administration of the Sacraments and Other Right and Ceremonies of the Church According to the Use of the Anglican Church of Canada*. Cambridge, England: Cambridge University, 1959.

Voices United: The Hymn and Worship Book of the United Church of Canada. Etobicoke, ON: The United Church Publishing House, 1996.

Wilkes, James. *The Gift of Courage*. Toronto, ON: Anglican Book Centre, 1979.

Woodman, Marion. *Bone: A Journal of Wisdom, Strength and Healing*. Toronto ON: Penguin Compass, 2001.

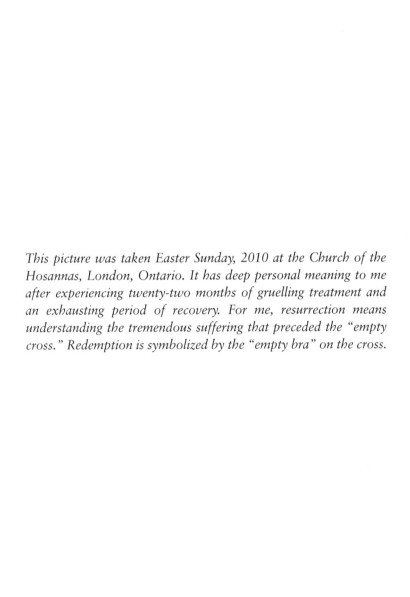

This picture was taken Easter Sunday, 2010 at the Church of the Hosannas, London, Ontario. It has deep personal meaning to me after experiencing twenty-two months of gruelling treatment and an exhausting period of recovery. For me, resurrection means understanding the tremendous suffering that preceded the "empty cross." Redemption is symbolized by the "empty bra" on the cross.

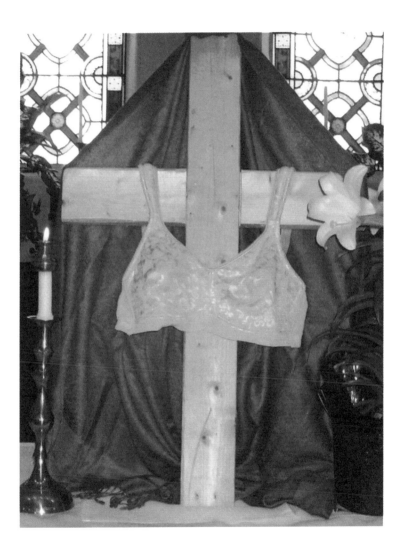

Notes